The WHOLE Method

Transform the WHOLE You from the Inside Out

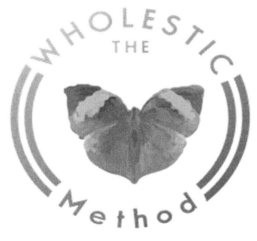

THE WHOLESTIC
Method
Transform the WHOLE You
www.debbiepotts.net

Debbie Potts

Debbie Potts

Published by Cardinal Rules Press
Cover design by uk.fiverr.com/Nisha
Edited and formatted by Marley Gibson
Interior Design and Formatting by AuthorsCrib.com

Although the author and publisher have made every effort to ensure the information in this book was correct at press time, the author and publisher do not assume and hereby disclaim any liability to any party for any loss, damage, or disruption caused by errors or omissions, whether such errors or omissions result from negligence, accident, or any other cause.

This publication is intended to provide helpful and informative material. It is not intended to diagnose, treat, cure, or prevent any health problem or condition, nor is it intended to replace the advice of a physician. No action should be taken solely on the contents of this book. The anecdotes and advice in this book are not intended as a substitute for the medical advice of physicians or healthcare professionals. Always consult your physician or qualified healthcare professional on any matters regarding your health and before adopting any suggestions in this book or drawing inferences from it.

Any and all product names referenced within this book are the trademarks of their respective owners. None of these owners have sponsored, authorized, endorsed, or approved this book. Always read all information provided by the manufacturers' product labels before using their products. The author and publisher are not responsible for claims made by manufacturers.

Printed in the United States.

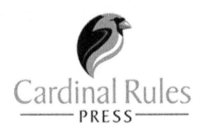

TABLE OF CONTENTS

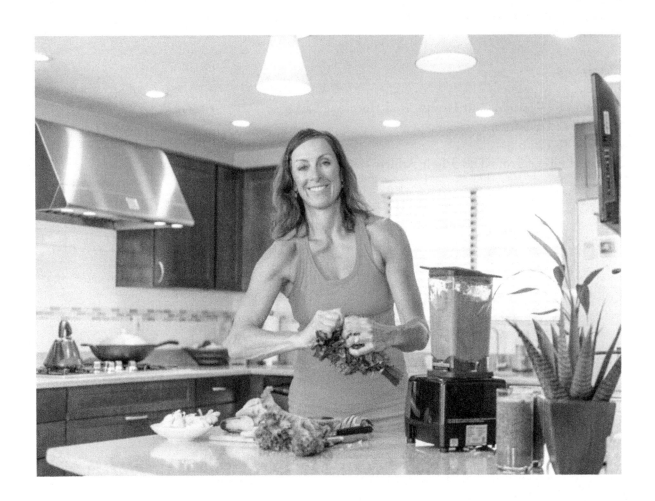

FOREWORD

This manual tells a story of a revolution that will transform our world and ourselves, one that has drawn together nutritionists, medical doctors, acupuncturists, chiropractors, scientists and psychiatrists in an unprecedented shift to addressing health from a systemic or "Wholestic" approach rather than from the reductionist diseases treatment paradigm that dominates Western healthcare.

An important takeaway is that we have been misled at best and lied to at worst about our most basic of health remedies, food. Who ever thought that spraying chemicals on our food was the right thing to do? Would you spray Roundup on your food before eating? Well, this is exactly what you are getting with most wheat products, factory farmed animals (they are fed the GMO sprayed grains) and non-organic foods. While genetic modification seems like a good idea, it has allowed big chemical companies to design products that boost their bottom line rather than actually help feed the world. It turns out that Roundup destroys your beneficial gut bacteria, not to mention has been deemed "a likely carcinogen" by the World Health Organization.

Great.

The misconception that fat, all fat, is bad for us has led to over processed edible food-like products that are full of sugar and other unpronounceable ingredients that have left our society fat and sick. In addition, our "busy addicted" society, whether created through sociological factors or through fake food-induced anxiety, has people short on time and eating out of boxes and fast food restaurants.

No Bueno.

To make matters worse, sleep deprivation has become a badge of honor. People actually brag about "only needing a few hours of sleep," that is until they crash and burn. Perhaps some people need a major collapse before they wake up and get some sleep.

One of the bottom lines of becoming healthy is reducing inflammation. Inflammation is implicated in just about every affliction including anxiety, depression, dementia (Alzheimer's), autism, heart disease and cancer. The SAD diet (Standard American Diet) is an inflammatory powerhouse, and that needs to change in order for our society to be healthy. I'm currently watching Dr. Mark Hyman's docu-series, *The Broken Brain.* While each episode talks about a different disease group, they all boil down to a common denominator: inflammation.

In the following pages, Debbie Potts will share what is considered the "state of the art" health information. Don't expect your doctor to understand any of this unless they are certified in functional medicine. These well-meaning doctors have been trained to treat disease (rather than promote health), usually through a prescription, and know little to nothing about nutrition. After Debbie's own "crash and burn" she is now not only talking the talk, she is walking the walk and helping others reach their full potential, from the inside out. This manual is a great start to a new you. I hope you benefit from this and share this new knowledge with your friends and loved one.

Ronda Collier
CEO and Co-Founder
SweetWater Health, LLC
www.BeatHealthy.com

Ronda Collier B.S.E.E., M.A., has more than twenty-five years of experience in high technology product development with a proven track record of delivering leading edge consumer electronic products within both privately held startups and Fortune 500 corporations. After graduating with a Masters in Holistic Psychology, she spent three years as an independent scholar researching non-invasive health monitoring techniques to improve overall personal well-being. This research led to the founding of SweetWater Health, L.L.C. in 2010.

PART ONE

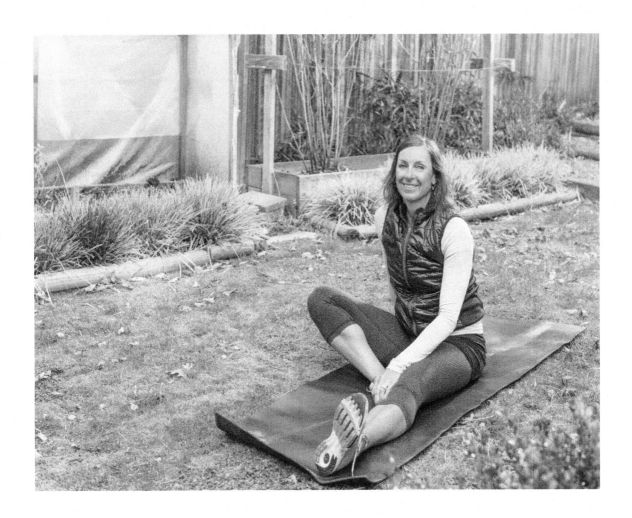

WELCOME TO THE WHOLESTIC
Method Manual

Welcome to The WHOLESTIC Method where you will learn to optimize your health, become a fat burner, and improve performance for life and sports.

Are you ready to start a new journey in life? The WHOLESTIC Method will take you down a different road to reach the optimal health you have been searching for. Most people have been looking for the "magic pill" to lose weight and improve performance and are shocked to discover there is no "magic pill," and change requires developing new habits and lifestyle choices.

Your journey here begins by learning the WHOLE body approach and then working on the WHOLE you. Through these pages, I will teach you how to become a fat-burning machine with less stress and better sleep.

The WHOLESTIC Method Sugar Detox and Reset Program is designed to put you on the right track toward healthy lifelong habits. You will learn how to balance your blood sugar levels by using fat, instead of sugar, as your main fuel source. In addition, you will have new tools to improve your sleep, lower your stress levels, and increase your strength and metabolism. Skin rashes, bloating and digestion issues will be a thing of the past.

It is important to understand that losing weight isn't only about exercising and making the right food choices. We must treat the body as a WHOLE, and this includes lifestyle choices such as "the busy epidemic," choosing to *respond* rather than *react* to adversity and getting the required 7-8 hours of *quality* sleep.

Together, we will delve into the eight key elements to improve your health by working on the WHOLE you. Western Medicine, with all its benefits, often treats the symptoms of the disease, masking the actual problem. In this manual, you will discover your WHY and treat the root cause of what's holding you back or limiting your performance.

Let's face it one size does not fit all and what works for one person may not work for another. Everyone is a unique being and The WHOLESTIC Method program is customized for you.

To be healthy involves a combination of elements that influence each other which is why I call it The WHOLESTIC Method. In the twenty-five years I have been a personal trainer, fitness instructor, triathlon/run coach, and a podcast host, I have discovered the definition of healthy doesn't mean you exercise two to three times per week. Based on my experience, to become a fat burner, reach optimal health, and gain peak performance in life and sports, we need to do more than workout a few times a week.

This program is based on my extensive experience which includes my observations and interactions with clients of all fitness levels, sizes, and ages. In these pages you will gain helpful tips and the tools to learn:

- The difference between being a sugar burner versus fat burner
- Eat for your metabolic type and be energized after you eat the right foods
- Various methods how to exercise efficiently and effectively
- Biohacking tips how to improve your quality of sleep
- Tips how to manage and lower your stress levels and triggers
- The importance of moving throughout the day and how
- Learn about digestion, leaky gut, gut health, and hormone balance
- How much clean water we should consume per day and why
- Why happiness matters, how to be grateful for each day and to add play into your life

Our society's belief that more is better, the shortest route is ideal, and that being busy all the time proves our success has led us down the path to less than optimal health. Creating a longer "health-span" requires a lifetime commitment. Keep up-to-date on new concepts with my podcast, The WHOLE Athlete, available on iTunes or my website (http://debbiepotts.net/) and via my latest book *Life is Not a Race*. For personal coaching, go to my webpage - http://debbiepotts.net/ and find the new client forms to get started.

Now that you are ready to take the deep dive into improving your health and well-being, let's get started.

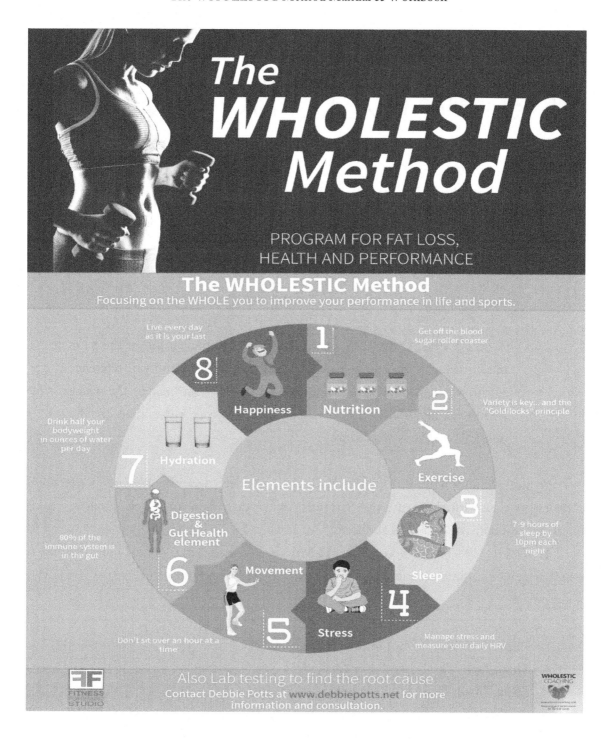

INTRODUCTION TO
The WHOLESTIC Method

I love the word WHOLE and the word HOLISTIC, so I created The WHOLESTIC Method program.

While the word "Holistic" is tossed around quite a bit these days, many people may not really understand what it means. Here are some definitions of Holistic:

ho·lis·tic

/h ōlistik/

Adjective PHILOSOPHY: characterized by comprehension of the parts of something *as intimately interconnected* and explicable only by reference to the whole. MEDICINE: characterized by the *treatment of the whole person*, taking into account mental and social factors, rather than just the physical symptoms of a disease.

Medical Definition of HOLISTIC: Relating to or *concerned with wholes or with complete systems* rather than with the analysis of, treatment of, or dissection into parts. Holistic medicine attempts to treat both the mind and the body.

The WHOLESTIC Method is designed with the knowledge that you are more than the sum of your parts and takes into account your mind, body, spirit, and environment. It eases you in via a 3 phase approach:

1. Phase One: The 5-Day Jumpstart Challenge
2. Phase Two: The 21-day Reset Challenge
3. Phase Three: The Maintenance 80/20 Program

Each phase consists of eight central elements which will be discussed in detail in the following chapters:

1. Nutrition

2. Exercise
3. Sleep
4. Stress
5. Movement
6. Digestion and Gut Health
7. Hydration
8. Happiness

Through my firsthand experience, I have learned that losing weight isn't about cutting calories and exercising more. I understand the body is interconnected and therefore, to get results, we need to look at the big picture from the inside out.

We are starting from the inside first as we need to adjust the mindset to create a positive attitude and lasting happiness. By working on building our foundation and creating goals, we establish new life-long habits and rituals. This new mindset will change our obsession with exercise as a means to lose weight and improve our health and overall performance. I am delighted you have decided to get off the hamster wheel and start this new journey in life.

Here are some of my secrets to success. Review these often or when you feel stuck:

- Get ready to make shift happen... get your mind right.
- Be ready to make changes by getting in right head space.
- Make the commitment to yourself, family, and friends.
- Set goals: Daily, weekly, and monthly.
- Keep the changes simple and stay focused.
- This is not a diet but a journey by creating new lifelong habits.
- Positive thinking; stop any negative programming.
- Keep a journal.

I know you can handle this challenge. I look forward to coaching you and observing your transformation. We will get you off the blood sugar roller coaster and on the road to becoming a fat burning machine.

Get started by reading this manual and then pull out your workbook to get begin on your personal journey.

We shall begin The WHOLESTIC Method journey by reviewing each of the eight elements in depth. The first element is Nutrition, which can be an entire book on its own, so we will cover the basics to get you started.

You can learn more on The WHOLE Athlete podcast.

ELEMENT #1
Nutrition

I n this chapter, we will explore the mechanics of metabolism and explain why fat is the preferred fuel source for our bodies. We will learn how to become a fat (versus sugar) burner and what fats to eat and what fats to avoid. We will talk about the current "fads" of intermittent fasting and ketogenic diets and will hear from experts on the optimal nutrition which includes healthy fats.

THE FAT MYTH

Contrary to the popular belief that fat and, particularly, saturated fat is bad for us, our bodies are actually designed to burn fat. The nutritional myth that fat is bad for us continues to fall apart as new studies emerge debunking the benefits of a low-fat diet. We have been brainwashed to believe eating natural saturated fats will increase our cholesterol, and high cholesterol leads to heart disease. Our obsession with fat has led to a dependence on non-fat and low-fat processed foods and has increased our consumption of carbohydrates, especially excessive amounts sugar hidden in every packaged manufactured food product.

The secret to health is eating nutrient dense, whole, nourishing foods are right for our metabolic type and keep our blood sugar levels balanced so we can be burning FAT instead of SUGAR for fuel.

Why are we taught to avoid fat and eat non-fat fake foods? Early theories assumed that the fat looking substance found in blocked arteries was caused by high cholesterol which was caused by eating too much fat. The Food Industry jumped on board to provide low-fat alternatives. The thing is, fat makes food taste good so they spent billions of dollars developing processed low-fat food that tastes good, and one of the primary ingredients to accomplish that was sugar or sugar derivatives. The new research indicates that small LDL particles (rather than regular LDL from your standard cholesterol test) combined with inflammation, is what is clogging the arteries. And guess what? The low fat processed food increases inflammation and may contribute to an increase in small LDL particles. The truth is:

1. We need fats as they provide a long burning source of energy (log versus kindling). We were designed to burn fat for fuel and can fast for periods of time.
2. We need fats as they act as building blocks for the cell membranes and hormones which our body is built up from cells and hormones regulate body functions.
3. We need fat to absorb fat soluble vitamins as A, D, E, and K.
4. We need fats for the proper use of proteins.
5. We need fats to protect the lining of our organs.
6. We need fats to help regulate energy absorption and slow the absorption fats of food rather than carbohydrates which are a quick energy source.
7. We need fat to feel full and satisfied, reduce cravings for bad fats, and empty calorie sugars.
8. We need fats to make food taste even better.
9. Quality sources of animal and tropical fats provide us with energy.
10. Good fats, as well as essential fatty acids, are required for optimizing our health as needed as the body doesn't make them.
11. Fats (besides the excess fat we store in our body) compose about fifteen percent (15%) of our body weight.
12. Fats are needed for blood clotting.
13. Fats are needed for muscle movement and endurance muscles.
14. Fats are needed for inflammation management- prostaglandin production (see my blog on this topic).

We need to eat fat to live, so let's stop being afraid to eat healthy natural fats. Eat fat to burn fat. Eat sugar to store fat.

FOOD AS NOURISHMENT

We often have a bond with food based on the time of day, stress, anxiety, or depression. Most of my clients who struggle with body weight often eat for various reasons besides being hungry or needing to fuel the body. We should try to think of food as nourishment for our system and fuel for our body that tastes amazing (if we actually focus on what we are eating and slow down enough to taste what we put in our mouths.) Food is sustenance as well as medicine for our body.

What is the definition of NOURISHMENT?

The food or other substances necessary for growth, health, and good condition: tubers from which plants obtain nourishment.

We need to learn how to enjoy *real* food that *nourishes* our body, mind, and soul. While the food we choose should keep us healthy and prevent most diseases, our society continues to depend on processed, man-made, factory, sugar-coated, vitamin-enriched, empty calorie foods to keep up with our fast-paced lifestyles. This is partially due to "the busy epidemic" (we believe we do not have time to prepare meals from whole food sources) and partially due to the addictive nature of these processed foods.

How is it that we do not make time to take care of our own health? We don't have time to eat right, to exercise, to move, or to sleep. What has happened to us? We are obsessed with the wrong things – we have plenty of time for checking our social media, text messages, and emails yet seem to have no time to throw an organic chicken in the oven and steam some broccoli.

Unbeknownst to us, these processed foods have modified our *microbiome*. The human digestive-tract contains trillions of microbes, known as the gut microbiome or gut flora, that form a symbiotic relationship with the rest of our WHOLESTIC selves. Microbiologists have known for some time that different diets create different gut flora. It turns out that part of the addictive quality of processed food is actually the bacteria in the gut craving the food. So, don't beat yourself up as you continue to crave your old favorites. Stick to your new food habits and the cravings will subside.

Please refer to my podcast, The WHOLE Athlete, to learn more:
- Breaking the fear of eating healthy fats
- Stop dieting by lowering calories
- Symptoms and causes of gut inflammation
- The myths of cholesterol, saturated fats, and heart disease

THE MECHANICS OF FOOD METABOLISM

Reality check; be honest with yourself: Are you consuming loads of carbohydrates, stressed out a lot and training at high heart rates for long periods of time in an attempt to burn off the calories? If so, you are probably burning sugar rather than fat as your main fuel.

Understanding the Sugar Roller Coaster and our Body

The blood sugar roller coaster, blood sugar dysregulation, and brain health are likely a priority for you or you would not be here. Wouldn't it be nice to be burning fat while we are sitting in the car, working, walking, and even when we are sleeping?

Why does our blood sugar go too low?

When we consume too many carbohydrates (especially without fat and proteins) and excess sugar, the digestive system breaks it down into sugar which enters the blood.

- As blood sugar levels rise, the pancreas produces insulin, a hormone that prompts cells to absorb blood sugar for energy or storage.
- As cells absorb blood sugar, levels in the bloodstream begin to fall.
- When this happens, the pancreas starts making glucagon, a hormone that signals the liver (which stores sugar as glycogen) to convert the glycogen into glucose and start releasing stored sugar.
- This interplay of insulin and glucagon ensure that cells throughout the body, and especially in the brain, have a steady supply of blood sugar.

As you can see we have a boomerang. Too much sugar or carbs spikes up the blood sugar levels. This requires the hormone insulin to lower the blood sugar levels and either transport it into the cells of the liver and muscles or move it to our fat stores. This leads to hypoglycemia when our blood sugar levels drop too low. Then, stored glucose, called glycogen, is converted back to glucose to increase blood sugar levels.

This constant boomerang of blood sugar levels is believed to be important in the development of type 2 diabetes. This means sugar spikes should be minimized in order to have a healthy metabolism.

Consequences of Low Blood Sugar

When your blood sugar drops too low, you have a blood sugar "crash" episode also known as hypoglycemia. When you experience that low blood sugar this "hangry" feeling manifest as:

- headache
- moody
- sugar craving
- impatience
- emotional
- hangry (hungry + angry = hangry)

We not only feel emotional and impatient, but we are also putting our body in emergency mode. Our blood sugar levels are too low, so the brain senses a crisis and must respond to the situation with an increased surge of glucose. The problem is the interpreted emergency signals the Hypothalamus to tell the Pituitary Gland to tell the Adrenal Glands to release the stress hormone cortisol to respond to the need for more glucose and to raise the blood sugar levels.

Goal to balance blood sugar levels and hormone insulin:
- Refined and processed carbohydrates
- Starchy foods and sugar
- Excessive consumption of high-glycemic carbohydrates = primary culprit in nutritionally caused health problems
- High glycemic carbohydrates = foods that raise blood sugar too rapidly. Example: rice, bread, candy, potato, sweets, sodas, and processed carbs.
- Processed carbohydrates=greatly increased glycemic index (measurement of their propensity to elevate blood sugar). Processing includes bleaching, baking, grinding, and refining foods.

- High-glycemic carbohydrates=causes inordinate insulin response. Chronic elevation of insulin leads to hyperinsulinemia, which has links to obesity, elevated cholesterol levels, blood pressure, mood dysfunction, etc.

Read the ingredients on food labels.

Your goal is to eat real food, so, ideally avoid eating food that is manufactured, includes a barcode, and has a long ingredient list.

When looking at food, ask yourself these questions:

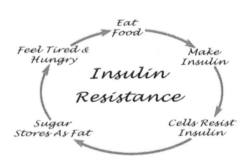

1. Are there less than five ingredients?
2. Do you know how to pronounce the ingredients?
3. Do you know the ingredients on the list?
4. Was the food around 10,000 years ago?
5. What to look for on the food label:
    a. Serving size and servings per container
    b. Total carbohydrates: total sugar
    c. Total Fiber

The macronutrient ratio: make sure you look at the back of the label to read ingredients that you understand but look at the ratio of protein to fats to carbohydrate (sugars and fiber, as well as the source on the label)

Another reason not to eat so much sugar every day... GLYCATION

Glycation is the process of excess glucose in the bloodstream that binds to protein or fat cells, and these sugar-coated molecules are distributed throughout the body creating "glycation," which is a form of "Cross-Linking". The sugar-coated protein molecules or cells lose their ability to communicate to other cells or within their own cells. The proteins, now "sticky" from excess sugar, then become cross-linked to other protein and DNA molecules. When these glycated molecules become hardened from cross-linking with other glycated molecules (glued together), the process is called AGES = Advanced Glycation End Products. The glycation damage could occur anywhere in the body as in our arteries, joints, and our cell membranes as they become hardened from the process of glycation...all a result of consuming excess sugar.

What is Cross-Linked?

Cross-linking occurs when a protein molecule becomes linked or connected to the other protein, sugar or lipid molecule. This makes the proteins stiff and hard. Think of bread that is soft and squishy and then in a few days, if left out on the counter; it becomes hard and stiff. It is a huge contributor to premature aging.

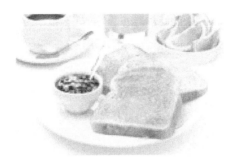

Beware of sugar hiding under different names such as fructose, high fructose corn syrup, brown rice syrup, molasses and cane juice to name a few. According to Dr. Mercola, "Fructose, in particular, is an extremely potent pro-inflammatory agent that creates AGEs and speeds up the aging process. It also promotes the kind of dangerous growth of fat cells around your vital organs that are the hallmark of diabetes and heart disease. In one study on fructose, sixteen volunteers on a controlled diet including high levels of fructose produced new fat cells around their heart, liver, and other digestive organs in just ten weeks."

Can glycation speed up the aging process of our skin?

Let's start with the definition of aging and how can we slow down the aging process. I know I want to slow down the wrinkles forming around my eyes.

A research paper in Dermato-Endocrinology by P. Gkogkolou *et.al.* says, "Aging is defined as the progressive accumulation of damage over time, leading to disturbed function of the cellular, tissue and organ level and eventually to disease and death. Aging is a complex, multifactorial process where genetic, endogenous and environmental factors play a role."

The conclusion from the study:

"There is ample evidence that AGEs play an important role in skin aging. There are also numerous studies investigating potential substances against excessive accumulation of AGEs in tissues. Some of these studies have already shown protective effects against diabetic complications. As controlled human studies investigating the effects of these anti-AGE strategies against skin aging are largely missing, this is a hot field for future research."

There are numerous studies in the National Institute of Health database called Pub Med. I encourage you to google this topic if you want to dig deeper.

The blood sugar roller coaster is not a ride you want to be on. It is time to get off. The excessive swing of going from one extreme to the other is stressful on the body – hyperglycemia to hypoglycemia (also known as dysglycemia). Plus, we are not only creating a sugar burning metabolism excellent at storing fat, but we are stressing the adrenals, slowing the thyroid, increasing the risk for insulin resistance, hormonal imbalances, and more problems as auto-immune disorders.

How do we balance our blood sugar levels throughout the day and get off the blood sugar roller coaster? We need to train our body systems to rely on fat for the main fuel source instead of depending on carbohydrates.

How do the organs work together to regulate blood sugar?

Our body has an innate intelligence that keeps our systems and processes in homeostasis, including keeping our levels of glucose in our bloodstream in ideal balance. Meet our blood sugar regulation management team: the Pancreas, the Liver, and the Adrenal glands. The goal is for us to do our part in keeping our blood sugar levels stable. This prevents overwork of the pancreas (which leads to insulin resistance). The same goes for the liver with the glucose-glycogen process as well as the adrenal glands cortisol process. High carb/high sugar diets can fatigue these organs and reduce the available amount of cortisol needed to raise blood sugar, resulting in hypoglycemia.

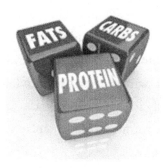

Food is energy. Let's review how we get fuel from the food we eat:

- Carbohydrates - simple sugars/starches, monosaccharides, glucose—bloodstream—storage as glycogen or fuel
- Fats - triglycerides, fatty acids—lymph system into blood—building blocks, fuel, and storage
- Proteins - amino acids, polypeptides—blood—building blocks and fuel

We only need so much glucose in our body at one time. When we have too much, glycogen (the stored form of glucose) is stored in the liver and muscles. Once the liver and muscles storage is at capacity, then the excess glucose gets shuttled to the fat cells by the hormone insulin. The brain is always working to monitor the blood sugar levels in our body to keep homeostasis and keep a slow stream of glucose in our blood. Due to poor diet, the average person takes in huge loads of sugar at once creating the "blood sugar roller coaster" ride.

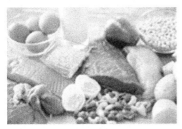
Most Americans eat a diet low in fat or high in rancid or hydrogenated fats.

On a cellular level, why is a poor or low-fat diet detrimental to health?

Lipids, or fats, include triglycerides, phospholipids, steroids, fatty acids, and fat-soluble vitamins (A, D, E, and K). Most fats get a bad reputation based on the "lipid hypothesis" which was proposed by researcher Ancel Keys. The "lipid hypothesis" was, or is to some people, a *theory* of the direct relationship between the amount of saturated fat and cholesterol in the diet to the incidence of coronary heart disease starting back in the 1950s. There is little evidence to support this theory, but to this day people are still confused and afraid to consume healthy fats, as well as the misunderstanding of what are healthy fats and essential fats.

Fat is essential to human health. Especially Essential Fatty Acids as Omega 3 fatty acids. Essential fatty acids cannot be made by the body, so we need to include them in our diet daily. Essential fatty acids may provide a protective effect against heart disease and strokes, decrease bone loss, reduced inflammation, promote wound healing, improve certain skin disorders, and improve mental functions.

Triglycerides are mainly saturated fats and found in meat, full-fat dairy sources and tropical plants of coconut, palm, and cocoa. At a cellular level, saturated fats play an important role in our body's chemistry. According to Sally Fallon, in "Nourishing Traditions," she explains:

- Cell membranes are approximately fifty percent (50%) saturated fatty acids
- Saturated fats give cells the stiffness and integrity to allow proper function
- Linolenic Acid = Omega 3 Fatty Acids
- Gamma-linolenic acid (GLA) is a long chain saturated fat is used to produce substances, as prostaglandins, localized tissue hormones, that regulate many processes at the cellular level
- Very long-chain fatty acids, as AA and DHA, are important to the function of the nervous system
- Phospholipids make up much of the cell membrane surrounding each cell
- Antimicrobial benefits from animal fats and tropical

Also, the obsession with low cholesterol has enriched Big Pharma who sell statins to millions of unsuspecting people (and statins have adverse side effects when taken for prolonged periods). We actually need cholesterol for cell membrane structure and stability. Cholesterol is a precursor to important corticosteroids, hormones to manage stress, and a precursor to producing our sex hormones. These are even more reasons to get current on the science of cholesterol as it is our natural healing substance to repair the damage from free radicals. Also, cholesterol is a predecessor to vitamin D, aids in the development of the brain and nervous system, and helps maintain the health of intestinal walls.

Today, the Standard American Diet (SAD) includes mostly polyunsaturated oils from commercial vegetable oils often derived from GMO soy and GMO corn. Instead, we should be consuming more naturally occurring fatty acids, saturated and unsaturated, from sources such as grass-fed butter, lard, tallows, coconut oil, and some olive oil. Mainstream media continues to scare people away from naturally occurring fats and create a fear of increased risk of heart disease. Dive into Sally Fallon's *Nourishing Traditions* book, and you won't be afraid of eating fat anymore.

Fat burning is a process called beta-oxidation. Fat metabolism takes places in the liver which converts fat into acetyl-coenzyme A, which through a complicated process is converted to energy for the cells in the form of ATP. It turns out that fat requires fewer steps than carbohydrates to create ATP and thus is a more efficient form of energy. Also fat gives us more energy as glucose = 36 ATP molecules as compared to fat molecules = 48 ATP molecules.

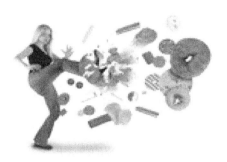

What about Ketosis and Ketones?

The ketogenic diet is not new. It may seem like a new trend or buzz word in the diet circles, but ketosis was developed in 1921 by a Dr. R. M. Wilder at the Mayo Clinic. Dr. Wilder developed the ketogenic diet to treat patients with seizures. Then, almost seventy years later, the concept reappeared again when someone else was searching for answers to help control seizures.

When deprived of carbohydrates, the liver becomes the sole provider or glucose, and once the liver is depleted of glycogen, it produces ketones. In summary:

- Ketones are a by-product of fat metabolism. The liver breaks down fat cells into fatty acids and ketones.
- The brain, muscles, and even the heart use water-soluble fats—or ketones—for energy.
- Ketones can work as fuel in the brain over glucose when needed.
- Saturated fats give cells the stiffness and integrity to allow proper function.

The main goal of the Ketogenic Diet is to burn, or rather metabolize, fat for fuel over sugar (glucose) which is also known as being in ketosis or being keto-adapted. Now, can we burn fat for fuel if we are not in ketosis?

Studies comparing different diet plans found that people can lose fat without being in ketosis. If your carb intake is too high, your body prioritizes burning these carbs first. You can promote fat burning by decreasing your carbohydrate intake, but you don't necessarily need to go as low as required to be in ketosis. Restrict your carbs slightly to help your body switch into fat-burning mode more easily.

When we are keto-adapted, we are using ketones (lipid-based fuel source) for our fuel source. When we rely primarily on using fatty acids and ketones for fuel, we can become more efficient fat burners, decrease body fat, and many health benefits as listed below. We can use fatty acids for fueling our muscles and ketones for use of other tissues especially the brain. One of the main signals of being in ketosis is the smell of acetone on your breath or in your urine since acetone can't be processed by the body, so it is excreted through our urine.

If we are not fat-adapted (those who eat a high carbohydrate diet), then when we are running low on fuel, we may hit the wall when running low on our carb fuel tank. Remember, we have 2,000 calories of carbs in the glycogen tank or, if we are fat-adapted, we can access 40,000 calories of fuel for energy.

Take note: each gram of glycogen is stored with around two grams of water, so we lose water weight when we begin our transformation from sugar burners to fat burners. Now, don't you want to be more metabolically efficient and burn fat for fuel?

GLYCEMIC INDEX

Remember, not all carbs are created equal. The Glycemic Index (GI) is a ranking or carbohydrates in foods according to how they affect blood sugar. You can check the GI of foods to help determine the best sources of carbohydrates:

According to the American Diabetes Association, the glycemic index (GI) is a ranking of carbohydrates on a scale from 0 to 100 according to the extent to which they raise blood sugar levels after eating. Foods with a high GI are those which are rapidly digested and absorbed and result in marked fluctuations in blood sugar levels. Low-GI foods, by virtue of their slow digestion and absorption, produce gradual rises in blood sugar and insulin levels and have proven benefits for health. Low GI diets have been shown to improve both glucose and lipid levels in people with diabetes (Type 1 and Type 2). They have benefits for weight control because they help control appetite and delay hunger. Low GI diets also reduce insulin levels and insulin resistance.

Recent studies from Harvard School of Public Health indicate the risks of ... Type 2 diabetes and coronary heart disease are strongly related to the GI of the overall diet. In 1999, the World Health Organization (WHO) and Food and Agriculture Organization (FAO) recommended that people in industrialized countries base their diets on low-GI foods to prevent the most common diseases... such as coronary heart disease, diabetes, and obesity.

To determine a food's Glycemic Index (GI) value, food containing 50 grams of carbohydrates are fed to people after an overnight fast, then their blood sugar levels are measured (finger prick) in fifteen to thirty-minute intervals over the next two hours. The blood samples are used to create a blood sugar response curve for the two-hour window post-consumption of the food. Don't worry; you don't have to do this to find the GI of your food, you can go online and easily find the GI for most popular items.

Some of you may try experimenting with a Ketogenic food plan, very high fat/low carb, for a few weeks or months, and then alternate mixing your ratios up by adding more vegetables for carbohydrates. Experiment with how you feel after eating (and pay particular attention to your energy levels) as you should be full for hours after a meal. Again, measure blood sugar levels and chart how you feel after eating. You should feel energized within twenty minutes of eating as well as satisfied (no sugar cravings) for over three hours for most people.

Remember not to give yourself a hall pass to eat unlimited amounts of food as people did with the Atkins Diet back when the book became a huge hit. You should feel full faster. Select good healthy fats, quality sources of protein, and non-starchy vegetables to feel comfortably full; not from a binge fest. We will go into detail on healthy fats later in this chapter.

Who should try Ketosis?

Long-term ketogenic diets are not for everyone, all the time. That said, it is being used medically with cancer patients to starve the cancer cells (which feed on glucose), for Neurological Diseases and for Obesity Weight Management

WEIGHT MANAGEMENT FOR OVERWEIGHT AND OBESITY

Blood sugar stabilization is key for prevention of weight gain, but also essential for prevention of common chronic disease. Living life with constantly elevated blood sugar levels places us at risk of multiple diseases (see www.chriskressor.com), and increases our risk of dying at an earlier age. When we eat primarily carbohydrates, we get on that pesky blood sugar roller coaster.

If you tend to have low blood sugar responses after a meal and then feel dizzy, anxious, shaky, and even confused, then you will benefit from balancing your blood sugar levels. A common cause of this reaction is when we have a meal too high in carbohydrates.

It took me years of doing my own research and self-experiment, as well as starting a podcast to learn about this concept. Why don't the mainstream media and others share this method? It could be that at the very top, the same people who profit from processed food also own the media companies. Take your health into your own hands.

When traditional medication and treatment doesn't work, then we often start searching elsewhere, and nutrition for healing and treating often comes into the picture. Nutrition is medicine as well as other natural remedies as essential oils.

Remember to experiment with how much fat, protein, and carbohydrates you need to stabilize your blood sugar and modify as needed. The results you want are to feel good, energized, and healthy from the inside out.

FIGHTING CANCER

Cancer cells feed on sugar. Cancer cells are not able to metabolize fat for their fuel like regular cells can. The reason people lose weight when they have cancer is because the cancer cells hog the blood sugar and starve the rest of the cells. The ketogenic diet has been shown to starve the cancer cells. I am so tired of too many friends and family members getting cancer when there are treatments available outside the allopathic western medicine paradigm. If I had cancer, I would go strictly ketogenic. That said, by balancing my blood sugar, I do not provide a ripe environment for cancer to get a foothold.

NEUROLOGICAL, BRAIN HEALTH, AND BRAIN-RELATED DISEASES

Alzheimer's, autism, ADHD, epilepsy-seizures, Parkinson's disease, ALS, stroke, dementia, and brain injuries all fall into the Neurological and Brain Health category. Did you know Alzheimer's disease is being termed Type-3 Diabetes now? I wonder if this increase in neurological diseases is related to the increase in sugar consumption in our country and the Standard American Diet (SAD) of processed high carbohydrate factory-made foods.

If you want to see amazing results from the Ketogenic diet for brain health, look up Dr. Mary Newport and Alzheimer's disease as well as Dementia. You will be sold on following a ketogenic diet for an alternative treatment.

When we start to have degeneration of the brain, we need to support the brain's nerve system. A diet high in healthy fats (around seventy percent (70%) has been shown to help the brain. If ketosis improves our ability to become fat-burning machines, we can also support our brain health when using ketones.

I shared earlier that the ketogenic diet has been used to treat epilepsy since the early 1900s. These days, more ketogenic specializing dieticians are using this diet for children suffering from seizures. I hope to see more research on kids with ADHD and ADD and the Ketogenic.

Other good resources and people to follow are Dr. David Pearlmutter (http://www.drperlmutter.com/) and Dr. Peter Attia (http://eatingacademy.com) for lots of research and success stories on using a low carb-high fat or ketogenic diet to treat neurological disorders as Parkinson's and Alzheimer's. They don't suggest this diet prevents these conditions; instead, they use a ketogenic diet is beneficial as part of the treatment plan.

There also may be benefits for those who suffer from depression or anxiety. Rather than taking anti-depressants, which is generally a long-term thing (think Big Pharma) perhaps doctors should look at mood related disorders and depression from a nutrition and diet perspective.

Summary: Benefits of a Ketogenic Diet?

The list is long, but just to offer a list of what current research supports the use of ketones for the following benefits:

- Weight loss
- Blood sugar balance and enhanced insulin sensitivity
- Increase satiety and decreased food cravings
- Improved energy levels, oxygen capacity, motor performance, and athletic performance
- Enhanced blood flow through vasodilation
- Migraine treatment
- Neuroprotective benefits in seizure disorders; ADHD; Alzheimer 's disease, memory, and cognitive function; Parkinson's Disease, Multiple Sclerosis
- Autism and improved behavior and social impacts
- Mood stabilization in bipolar disorder (type II)
- Stroke prevention; cardiovascular disease; metabolic syndrome management; improved cholesterol levels
- Inflammation management
- Endurance enhancement

Learn more about the benefits of Ketosis for the brain and more benefits...

- http://tinyurl.com/MariaMindBodyHealth
- http://tinyurl.com/DietDoctorLowCarb
- http://tinyurl.com/EffectsLowCarbDiet
- http://tinyurl.com/BrainKetones
- The Ketogenic Diet by Maria Emmerich
- Keto Clarity by Jimmy Moore
- The Art and Science of Low Carbohydrate Performance by Volek and Phinney
- The Art and Science of Low Carbohydrate Living by Volek and Phinney
- http://thewholesticmethod.pruvitnow.com/resist-the-dark-side-and-easily-shift-into-ketosis/

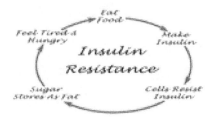

HOW DO YOU BECOME A FAT BURNER?

In order to become a fat burner, you must change the way you eat and eat for your metabolic type. You don't have to eat an extremely low carb diet forever but you do need to re-train your body how to choose its preferred source of fuel: fat.

Recall that the main macronutrient to activate the fat *storing* hormone insulin is carbohydrates. Some carbohydrates are obviously better choices than other and are preferably consumed with healthy fats and a protein to balance the blood sugar levels. If we focus on the balance of our blood sugar levels, we can help keep our insulin release low and ideally promote increased fat oxidation and decrease fat storage.

Lord Kelvin said, "If you cannot measure it, you cannot improve it." By measuring our blood sugar after meals, we adjust our diets to become fat burning machines. I have been testing my blood sugar levels (and eventually ketone levels) for years. I use the same device diabetics use daily to monitor their blood sugar levels.

You can do the same. Measure your blood sugar levels two hours after you eat to make sure you ate the right amount of macronutrients for your metabolic type. If correct your blood sugars will stabilize, you will burn fat for fuel, and possibly lead you to ketosis (if going low carb and even supplementing with products as Prüvit). Check out my shopping links on my web page www.thewholesticmethod.com for my favorite glucose and ketone level testing kits. Also, see my podcast on Metabolic Typing.

I find it not only interesting, but eye-opening to measure my blood sugar levels after eating, and you will too. My health is important to me, so knowing what I choose to eat and how my body will respond is a priority to me.

What about Intermittent Fasting?

If you have been listening to podcasts for a long time, you know about Jimmy Moore. When you have questions about low carb, ketosis, and fasting, he is the man. Jimmy has been immersed in low-carb eating for years now and is the author of many books including a new one on fasting and is the one behind the Livin' La Vida Low-Carb fame.

Jimmy Moore shared with me: "I was originally extremely skeptical of the idea of intermittent fasting. It didn't make sense to me to allow yourself to go hungry for some mysterious benefits to your health. But, once I began eating a low-carb, moderate protein, high-fat, ketogenic diet, I found it was natural to spontaneously fast for upwards of 18-24 hours without really thinking about it. With my history of eating a lot of food that led me to once weigh in at over 400 pounds, it's a miracle I now only eat about one to two meals daily. The synergistic blend of keto with fasting is a recipe for incredible, robust health like you've never experienced before."

Dr. Mercola, of the famed www.mercola.com—the World's #1 Natural Health website—talks often about what science says about intermittent fasting to maintain your ideal body weight, have more energy, and feel great. Many research articles suggest fasting occasionally to improve health and longevity especially if you are struggling with weight issues. Note that most Religions have some level of fasting built into their rituals. The founders of the Religions knew something. Intermittent fasting helps switch you from being a sugar burner to a fat burner and has additional cleansing effects.

No one is suggesting you starve yourself as this can lead to binging after the fast. By gradually adding in periods of fasting, we can train our bodies to become fat adapted by encouraging our body's manufacturers of the fat burning enzymes. As we become fat adapted, we are down-regulating the enzymes that burn carbohydrates. I have clients who eat one main meal for the day, ideally in the afternoon or early evening depending on their work and family schedule.

Dr. Mercola and other fasting experts suggest the fast must be at least sixteen hours to be the most effective in becoming fat adapted. Also, it takes your body about six to eight hours to metabolize glycogen stores before shifting to burning fat. Therefore, don't refuel your glycogen stores before that time period (eight hours) or you will have more of a challenge activating the fat burning enzymes.

Remember, to start adding in intermittent fasting gradually if you are going to experiment or do the 5-Day Jumpstart Challenge. It is a gradual process, so start by not eating after dinner, then see if you can wait until lunch to eat.

EXPERT OPINIONS

Next, let me share some of the opinions from various guest hosts on my podcast, The WHOLE Athlete.

As I continue to research intermittent fasting, low carb-high fat eating, "no sugar no grains" (from Vinnie Tortorich termed as NSNG) and the ketogenic diet, I become more aware of how carbohydrate dependent our society has become. Most Americans are addicted to sugar and dependent on manufactured factory foods (Franken-foods). Our body knows how to digest, breakdown, and assimilate real food, but when you empty garbage into your mouth, it's no wonder we have so many health problems in our society. Vinnie Tortorich keeps it simple as he teaches his clients and podcast followers his "No Sugar-No Grains" philosophy. If we gain a better understanding of what is good to eat (and why) and then focus on the abundance of good foods, we can choose to create amazing tasting meals and stop dwelling and focusing on foods that compromise health.

LAURA KUNCES

I have interviewed Laura Kunces, Ph.D., R.D., a Nutrition expert from EXOS which is a well-known training organization for elite and professional athletes. Part of their platform focuses on training people from the inside out. We agreed that science has changed over the last few decades and we can only do so much with exercise and strength training. The type of foods we are eating makes a difference, but it is never a one size fits all solution. We are all different with unique gut microbiomes. A calorie is not always an equal calorie: 100 calories of broccoli versus the same calories of ice cream are obviously not the same quality source of nutrition, and our bodies handle those calories quite different.

Laura says before you go to the doctor for gut irritation, look at ways you can isolate and identify the cause of your problem yourself. She talks about what she calls an "elimination diet." This is the purging of obvious offenders from your diet. Give it a couple of weeks, and then slowly start reintroducing food items one at a time. This lets you identify the specific substance causing your irritation, rather than immediately taking antibiotics, which could make the situation worse. You can also try the Bulletproof Food detective app to discover foods that you are sensitive to.

Like many previous guests on my podcast, Laura emphasized the importance of real food. This was one thing that can particularly affect athletes since it is fashionable to workout with energy drinks or other simple sugars and carbohydrates. In addition, athletes are creatures of habit and may have gotten into a real rut with how they eat. We too may have become in the habit of eating particular items before, during or after a workout, items that may or may not be good for our health goals.

We will get into gut health in the digestion chapter, but do you know how your diet impacts your gut health? More research continues to come out into mainstream media about our good and bad gut bacteria. We need to optimize the bacteria ratio so we can impact how we absorb and utilize nutrients in our body. Common gut issues such as irritable bowel syndrome and bloated bellies are increasing in athletes as they make poor nutrition choices. Probiotics are always suggested as well as lots of green vegetables, fermented foods, and drinks. Prebiotics are foods for the good bacteria - probiotics are good bacteria.

Laura Kunces suggests boosting our immunity by improving gut health. We need to inspect our poop (read about THE POOPY POLICE by Paul Chek ☺) and get lab testing. Gluten and grains can cause gut health issues, as well, even for athletes. A low-carb-high-fat food plan seems to be best for gastrointestinal issues for most endurance athletes of all levels.

I asked Laura to list five foods we should include in our diet plan for endurance athletes. She said:

1. Eggs – including the yolk (note that this is also a culprit for many people)
2. Raw mixed nuts – almonds, cashews, pistachios, and macadamia nuts (not coated with sugar)
3. Cheese – satiating and good for cravings (try raw goat or sheep cheese)
4. Dark chocolate – read the label for sugar content and get the low sugar bar
5. Mixed berries (organic)

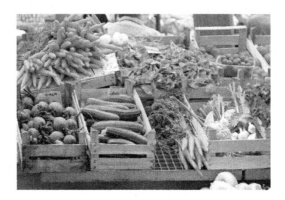

Many, ahem, most people think a calorie is a calorie and to lose weight we count what goes in and what is burned. This is simply not true. It's far more complex as you have learned in this chapter.

While you may lose weight using the calorie in, calorie out school of thought, a more sustainable approach is to consider exactly what you're eating and how it affects your body. More specifically, how it affects your gut (or microbiome) and what your gut is actually absorbing.

All calories aren't created equal because they impact our internal processes—metabolism, insulin stimulation, energy stores, and more—differently. With this in mind, the old saying of eat less, work out more should be something more like, "eat foods that are ideal for your system."

Whether you're trying to gain muscle, lose body fat, gain body weight, or a combo, step one is figuring out your current body composition. Learning about your body composition and knowing your percentages of fat, bone, water, and muscle is a great starting point and a terrific barometer of your health and fitness. Tracking it, along with factors like strength, mood, productivity, and sleep, will help you gauge the effectiveness of your training and nutrition program. You may even be able to quantify an ideal body composition range at which you feel and perform best. Thankfully, science has helped develop numerous assessment tools. Which method is best for you?

You can get in touch with Laura at *lkunces@teamexos.com*. Find out more about EXOS at www.exosfuel.com.

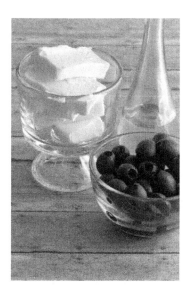

DR. CATE SHANAHAN

Another knowledgeable expert is Dr. Cate Shanahan. Dr. Cate is a board-certified physician, but she has some unorthodox views on nutrition. As she says, her focus on nutrition, as opposed to pharmaceuticals, is becoming more common in the medical community, but there is still a long way to go. She has written two books on dieting called D*eep Nutrition* and *Food Rules.* She is also the medical director of The Fat Burn Factory.

Dr. Cate says doctors are blasted with the same sort of information the general public has. For example, pushing the idea of fruits and vegetables as a kind of mantra for health is not necessarily the best nutrition. She points out that fruits and vegetables are extremely different in that fruits are often packed with sugars. Vegetables are often high in essential nutrients and low in sugar, but they are treated as equivalent or even lesser than fruits.

However, she's still mystified as to why this approach to treatment is still largely unrecognized. It follows scientific knowledge, so the fact that it is still somewhat underground

The WHOLESTIC Method Manual & Workbook

doesn't make sense. Unless, of course, you consider that most MDs have a grand total of two weeks' nutrition training in medical school and a whole lot of training on prescription drugs. I suggest ordering Dr. Shanahan's new book and follow her to keep up with cutting-edge nutrition research from a medical doctor who thinks outside of the box.

TERI MOSEY

Teri Mosey came on my podcast to talk about nutrition and natural foods after I listened to her presentation at the IDEA World Fitness Convention. I liked what she had to share, especially to fitness trainers from around the world. Teri Mosey uses a unique way of blending traditional Chinese alternative medicine with western philosophies to develop her approach to medical and nutritional strategies. Her approach is to emphasize using the nutrition in food as medicine as well as sustenance. It is also an integrated approach to the body, including the interaction of various hormones. This is quite different from the Western Medicine training that treats each organ, cell, molecule, and disease as being separate from the whole you.

Teri talks about the way we eat and how it needs to fit us as individuals so we don't need to eat at exact times or only eat specific things for particular meals. For example, eggs aren't only for breakfast. She recommends having soup for breakfast. It's socially accepted rules that require us to eat specific foods at set times. For the same reasons, she refrains from recommending joining what she calls the "tribes of eating." This dedication to a kind of diet glosses over individual dietary needs, so keeping your diet varied and don't adhere to an arbitrary set of rules. Going your own way will serve you better nutritionally.

What she does advocate is natural food because it will be a better choice no matter who you are. Especially in the United States, it isn't necessary for us to eat foods packed with preservatives and other chemicals. For many of us, there's an abundance of organic real food available, and natural foods are easy to get most of the time. You don't need to plan for food to last for months or years on your shelf.

Teri points out that seventy percent (70%) of the immune system is associated with the digestive system. Throughout the different seasons, people get sick for different reasons. Often, it's the kids going back to school and bringing home all the germs they pick up, but a healthy immune system developed from a good diet will be able to fight off even the toughest germs.

Teri makes it clear there is less of a division between body and mind than generally accepted. Thus, stress on the mind will certainly result in clear consequences for the body and training. She states we aren't simply physical beings and our nature is mental, spiritual, and physical.

Athletes are especially prone to the kind of simplification that leads to a nutritional imbalance through too much exercise. Her approach to nutrition is also very important and emphasizes the value of a varied diet. Athletes can get focused on a few, specific types of food as easily as they get preoccupied with a single type of hormone.

She also says that body detoxification is happening all the time. You can help this along with the proper diet. Overall, Teri emphasizes the importance of balance and a holistic approach to all aspects of our life.

Teri Mosey has twenty years' worth of experience as a consultant, educator, exercise physiologist, and natural chef. Her knowledge and expertise have developed over the years to include studies of Eastern and Western philosophies, energy medicine, and culinary exploration.

MARIA EMMERICH

I did a podcast episode (#69) of *The WHOLE Athlete* with Maria Emmerich, bestselling author and wellness expert in nutrition and exercise physiology. I asked her what she thinks the Top Ten Weight Loss Mistakes are:

1. Using nuts, nut flours, seeds, psyllium (a form of fiber made from the husks of the Plantago ovata plant's seeds) for weight loss – DO NOT SUBTRACT FIBER
2. Consuming dairy
3. Drinking calories, including Bullet Proof coffee
4. Eating when you are not hungry
5. Consuming alcohol
6. Not enough sleep
7. Eating too much protein
8. Damaged liver
9. Eating before bed and exercising at the wrong time of day
10. Adrenal fatigue and stress

In her book, *Keto-Adapted*, Maria says "When I read about how you need to eat every two to three hours to fuel your metabolism and muscles, I find it so ridiculous. Sure, if you are a sugar burner, you will need to eat that often, not only because you are hangry, but because eating a high-carbohydrate diet burns up amino acids so you need insulin to increase muscle. But if you eat a well-formulated keto-adapted diet, it spares protein from being oxidized and therefore preserves muscle. Branched-chain amino acids (BCAA) are considered essential because your body can't make them, so you need to consume them for proper muscle building and repair (as well as for replenishing red blood cells). What I find so interesting is that BCAA oxidation rates usually rise with exercise, which means you need more if you are an athlete. However, in keto-adapted athletes, ketones are burned in place of BCAA. Critics of low-carb diets claim that you need insulin to grow muscles; however, with a well-formulated keto-adapted diet, there is less protein oxidation and double the amount of fat oxidation, which leaves your muscles in place while all you burn is fat." She also adds "Breakfast isn't the most important meal of the day... breaking your fast is."

DR. MERCOLA

Dr. Mercola did his research and put it together into an article, sharing his ideas on how to slow down the aging process. His thoughts are similar to my The WHOLESTIC Method eight elements, and then some.

A key overlooked issue is adding stress management to the mix (see more tips on The WHOLE Athlete podcast and in The WHOLESTIC Method manual chapter on Stress). Stress is related to inflammation as the stress response activates the adrenal glands, and they are part of the anti-inflammatory process. If the adrenal glands are fatigued, then the body may experience more inflammation (hypoadrenia). It is extremely important for people to learn how to slow down, relax and unwind. Some will gravitate toward meditation and yoga, others will prefer walking, and others will choose prayer. These activities, along with a positive mental state can activate the Parasympathetic Nervous System (PNS) which balances the Sympathetic Nervous System (SNS) also known as "Fight or Flight."

A few more pointers include:
- Eat more whole foods lower carbohydrate (more vegetables), moderate protein (grass-fed sources), and higher healthy fats (especially add essential fatty acids - another blog to come on EFA).

- Get outside more often in daylight for your Vitamin D for safe sun exposure or take a good source of oral vitamin D with fish oil (recommended by Dr. Axe).
- Add more omega 3 fatty acids such as krill oil, fish oil, and good sources of essential fatty acids (see another blog on EFA).
- Get your antioxidants from whole foods.
- Add coconut oil into your cooking and foods, as well as in skin products (check my DIY gifts on Pinterest).

I continue to investigate how we can burn fat for fuel, become fat adapted, and become more metabolically efficient at rest and during exercise. New research continues to be released on the ketogenic diet as well as the benefits of being in ketosis. I am interested in learning more about how we can burn fat as our main fuel without having to go super low-carbohydrate to be in ketosis. Prüvit is a company that created ketone supplements and provides an easier way to obtain the benefits of Ketosis without having to eat as low of carbohydrate diet.

Get your mind right while you curb sugar cravings and feel fuller longer; find out for yourself. Measure your blood sugar levels or even ketone levels daily for thirty days to discover how your body reacts to sugar. Remember, our goal is to balance the blood sugar levels.

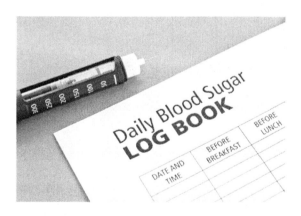

HEALTHY FATS

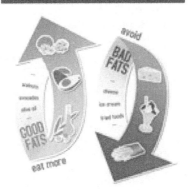

Healthy fats, unhealthy fats, which is which? We get so much conflicting information that we often throw up our hands and go for the GMO Canola oil-drenched fries.

In general, a good source of fats includes:
- Monounsaturated fats: olive oil, peanut oil, canola oil, avocados, and most nuts, as well as high-oleic safflower and sunflower oils.
- Polyunsaturated fats: soybean oil, corn oil, fatty fish like salmon, mackerel, herring, and trout.

Fats we want to stay away from include:
- Industrial made trans-fats: the process of hydrogenation of fats takes healthy oils into solids.
- Partially hydrogenated oils.

There are several different classes of fats including Polyunsaturated fat, Monounsaturated fat, Saturated fat and Trans fat. Essential Fatty Acids are a type of Polyunsaturated fat necessary for human body and must be included in the diet.

Why Do We Need to Include Essential Fatty Acids (EFAs) in our Diet?
- **EFAs**, are fats that are required for health that body does not make itself. Therefore, we must get these fats from our diet.
  - Linoleic Acid: Omega 6 Fatty Acids

- Alpha Linolenic Acid: Omega 3 Fatty Acids
- **Prostaglandin (PG)** production is formed from elongated EFAs and these hormone-like substances are needed by nearly all body tissues and fluids in the body. Their functions include cell communication system, helping with homeostasis, blood flow in kidneys and *controlling inflammatory function.*
- Specific Prostaglandins are named with a letter and a number, such as PG1, PG2, PG3. Each specific PG has a different role in the inflammatory process. – For example PG1 and PG3 anti-inflammatory and PG2 are pro-inflammatory.

Most people are deficient in fat... or rather deficient in the fatty acids required to help with prostaglandin formation to aid in the inflammatory process in the body.

Polyunsaturated fats:

From a chemical standpoint, polyunsaturated fats are simply fat molecules that have more than one unsaturated carbon bond in the molecule. Oils that contain polyunsaturated fats are typically liquid at room temperature but start to turn solid when chilled. Olive oil is an example of a type of oil that contains polyunsaturated fats. Polyunsaturated fat is found in vegetable oils and seafood and includes the EFAs omega-3 and omega-6 fatty acids.

While vegetable oil is polyunsaturated, be mindful of GMO soy and corn oils as they are in everything. GMO corn is modified with a gene that breaks open the stomach of insects and kills them. These "BT" toxins are found in most people and are linked to a plethora of diseases. The GMO soy is no better.

- Omega-3 fatty acids are found in: fatty fish such as salmon, mackerel, and sardines, flaxseeds, walnuts
- Omega-6 fatty acids are found in: corn, safflower, peanut and most oils (LINOLEIC ACID)
  - GLA = Gamma Linolenic Acid = Black Current Seed, Evening Primrose Oil, and Borage Oil
  - DGLA = Dihomo-gamma-linolenic Acid

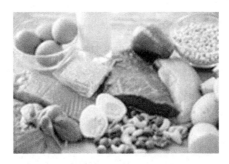

Saturated fats:

Saturated fat is solid at room temperature and is mostly in animal foods such as milk, cheese, and meat. It is also found in tropical oils such as coconut oil, palm oil, and cocoa butter. I recommend staying away from (like never eat) margarine and shortening and only use grass-fed butter like Kerry Gold.

Trans fats:

Trans fat is a fat that has been hydrogenated, a process that increases shelf life and makes the fat even harder at room temperature. While this makes crispier crackers and flakier pie crusts, it is extremely bad for you, so avoid it at all costs. Thankfully, Big Food has jumped on the "No Trans Fat" bandwagon, though be mindful when purchasing processed foods, particularly chips, crackers, and cookies.

Plus, we have four other types of fatty acids that are known to be "conditionally essential":

1. GLA: gamma-linolenic acid
2. AA: arachidonic acid
3. EPA: eicosapentaenoic acid
4. DHA: docosahexaenoic acid

Which Fat for What?

We have different types of fat available to eat and cook with but which ones are the best to use? Most fats are a combination but referred to the primary type of fat.

Saturated fats:
- The most stable to cook with
- Animal fats and tropical oils
- Solid at room temperature

- Non-essential fat as body can make these fats
- Does not go as rancid as easily
- Source: coconut oil, lard

Monounsaturated fats:
- Relatively stable- cooking at low temperature as a sauté
- Liquid at room temperature
- Non-essential fat as body can make these fats
- Sources: olive oil, almonds, cashews, and avocados

Polyunsaturated fats:
- Relatively unstable - not to cook with and very fragile – never heat them or else you take a healthful oil and rob the healthy properties converting it into unhealthy oil
- These fats go rancid easily so buy in quantities you will use quickly
- Chemically altered if used in prepared foods (hydrogenation)

NEXT... A new fuel for your brain: MCT Oil

We keep hearing about using MCT oil for weight loss and brain fuel. Bullet Proof coffee anyone? But, do you know anything about MCT oil?

To dive deeper into the world of MCT oil and brain fuel, I did a podcast episode with my guest co-host, Brock Armstrong, who worked with Ben Greenfield specializing in Ketosis and bio-hacking techniques. He now works full-time for Dave Asprey who created the well-known Bullet Proof coffee and popular bestselling book, *The Bulletproof Diet.*

What is MCT Oil?

MCT oil is basically a concentrated form of coconut oil. Coconut oil contains what are called Medium Chain Triglycerides (MCT) and that produce a plethora of health benefits. Because your body sends MCTs directly to your liver, this oil is excellent for instant energy. It also provides other benefits including brain health and weight loss. It is quickly metabolized for energy and easily digested.

The interest in MCT oil has grown over the recent years partially due to the well-known benefits of coconut oil as well as by a well-known study by Dr. Mary Newport. Dr. Newport used coconut oil to treat her husband's advancing Alzheimer's and I strongly encourage you to check this out. You can find her articles and videos at http://coconutketones.com.

Why do we want MCT Oil in our diet when we are taught that fats, especially saturated fats, cause high cholesterol and heart disease? The information in the mainstream media is conflicting and outdated and we must consider who is funding the research. Big Food companies have spent a fortune developing addictive tasty food like substances that will have a long shelf life. Big Pharma makes a fortune off of you once you get sick from the processed foods. Together they do not want you being satiated and healthy.

Why take MCT oil? It depends on your use...

Like other saturated fats, you can use coconut oil for cooking at higher heat. If you need to fire up the brain or required quick energy for sports performance, then go directly to the source and add some directly to your coffee, tea or smoothie, or make use it in your salad dressing or anywhere else you use oil. How much? Studies suggested a range of 5 to 70 grams of MCT oil daily. If your goal is for overall good health, then just use coconut oil daily.

Digestion of MCT oil:
- Rapidly broken down and absorbed in the body
- MCTs go directly to the liver and used as instant energy or turned into ketones
- MCT oils are less likely stored as fat as they are more rapidly broken down and absorbed into the body than most often used as fast energy source over glucose (when combined with a low-carb diet)

Benefits of adding MCT oils to low-carb food plan:
- Improves blood sugar regulation and insulin sensitivity (Type 2 diabetes benefits)
- Improves metabolism
- Improves appetite regulation
- Beneficial for treating many health issues as seizures, Alzheimer's, and dementia
- May improve cholesterol levels and higher antioxidant vitamin levels
- Improved brain function as MCT oils produce ketones
- Improved learning, memory, and brain processing (those with APOE4 gene)

Sources of MCT oil:

- Coconut oil – greater than 60% = 4 types of MCT, 50% Lauric acid/C12 and smaller amounts of capra fatty acids C6, C8, and C10. Best natural sources of MCT oil.
- Palm kernel oil – greater than 50%
- Dairy products - 10-12% = 4-12% Capra fatty acids (C6, C8 and C10) and 2-5% of Lauric acid (C12)
- 100% Caprylic Acid C8
- 100% Capric Acid C10
- Or combination of C8 and C10

Remember to be aware of where your food came from especially animal sources... Is it wild caught fish? Grass-fed beef? Or, is it factory produced grain-fed animal source from feedlots? Farmed fish are lower in omega 3 fatty acids than wild fish and have usually been treated with antibiotics to ward off sea lice. Go wild, go grass fed and go organic.

A critical factor to remember is that for the body to absorb fats, proper digestion is required. Fat malabsorption, also called steatorrhea, is the inability to properly digest fats. This can be caused by liver congestion, poor quality bile (gall bladder issues) and lack of a pancreatic enzyme (lipase). This is why a WHOLESTIC approach is required for optimal health.

The big five WHOLESTIC Method Top 5 Nutrition tips for becoming a fat burner:

1. _____
2. _____
3. _____
4. _____
5. _____

The WHOLESTIC Method to improving fat loss, health and performance for life and sports by working from the inside out

Element #2
Exercise

We all know we need to exercise two to three times per week especially as we age. It makes our bones stronger, improves our posture, and mends our metabolism. Many people exercise to burn fat and lose weight without knowing which exercise is the best for their goals.

Houston we have a problem – Most people either don't exercise consistently or they do it too much. Not only should exercise be a daily habit such as brushing your teeth, it should be fun, provide energy, make you laugh and puts a smile on your face. Exercise should be your play time, not something you dread.

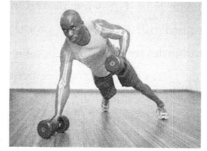

People often give up on exercising weekly because of boredom and monotony. I would get so bored if I went to the gym four days a week to do the elliptical and stationary bike while reading or watching a TV show. Plus, you don't get many benefits from doing only stationary cardio machines. Yes, you do get some credit for moving and getting your cardiovascular benefits (if you get your heart rate up to your aerobic zone or do intervals) however you don't get the full benefits that you can achieve by mixing in resistance training, outdoor nature visits, and yoga. Most people I see who are doing indoor cardio equipment are reading the newspaper or doing crossword puzzles. While this is better than sitting on the sofa, there is huge room for improvement.

Also, some people exercise like crazy and still don't achieve their weight loss goals. It isn't due to a lack of trying or wanting, they are simply not exercising the most effective and/or efficient way. From my experience, one of the top reasons people fail at sticking with an exercise program is because they try to do it *alone* and do the same thing every time.

EXERCISE AS A FUN HABIT

How can you make exercise a habit and part of your lifestyle? My suggestion is to first take a hard look at your usual schedule and find a time that will work *consistently*. Many people use the "I'm too busy" excuse as they complain about needing to exercise while enjoying happy hour at the local pub. I'm not saying you can't do happy hour. I am saying to take an honest look at your activities and find a place in your day for exercise. For some it is before work, others go to the gym or for a walk/run at lunch and others prefer after work. I recommend adding the exercise to your calendar and scheduling other activities around it.

Once you know you have time slots committed, surround yourself with other people in shared workouts. This can be shared personal training sessions (thirty minutes is ideal), group training sessions or classes a few days per week. Gather some friends for regular evening and/or weekend hikes or bike rides. If dancing is your thing, find a Zumba class nearby that fits your schedule. The key is to find a group that makes you feel like part of a community. This will help motivate you to show up (or else your workout partners will be giving you a hard time). Once you meet new workout friends, you will hold yourself to a higher standard as others will be looking to you for support while also holding you accountable. You will enjoy going just to see your friends and experience the community.

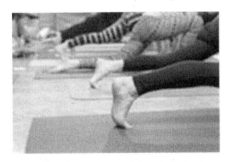

After twenty-five years in the fitness industry, and as a competitive athlete myself, I see all our clients work harder when matched with other workout friends. They not only work harder, but they are more consistent with their workouts, more focused, and more motivated when in a group. The outcome is that our clients achieve the results they have been striving for over the years that they did not achieve by working out alone in the big box gyms.

Another reason people don't stick with an exercise program is they make it boring and repetitious. They do the same workout every session. I believe in mixing up the type and style of workout sessions, including indoor and outdoor play sessions, MAF (Max Aerobic Function Heart Rate) style heart rate training, heavy strength training days, high-intensity interval, and mobility days, as well as restorative yoga, Pilates, and movement training sessions. At my studio, I created a mixed workout training schedule so each day our clients are doing a different type of workout and training with MYZONE heart rate monitors to monitor intensity, effort level and to avoid overtraining. To train your body to become a better fat burner at rest and during exercise we need to:

1. Lift heavy weights
2. Train by heart rate
3. Avoid the black hole (training in one zone above aerobic heart rate)
4. Work-in as much as your work-out (focus on inside and outside)

As a longtime trainer, I have heard all the stories there are to hear. Many people come up with what are, quite frankly, excuses rather than reasons for quitting their fitness program after only four weeks:

- Lack of enjoyment... boring.
- No time, or so they say (at the pub, glass of wine in hand ☺).
- Unrealistic expectations, quick results, or else.
- The wrong kind of motivation from a trainer or coach, overtraining without foundation built.
- Fear of pain or lack of experience; a qualified experienced coach is key.
- Poor atmosphere, equipment, cleanliness, and access, so select the ideal workout studio for your personality and to meet your expectations or else you probably won't stay long.
- Lack of structure and/or support. If you don't feel support and encouragement from your coach and training partners, you will be discouraged and unmotivated to continue training.

For this reason, we at Fitness Forward Studio have built up an amazing community. We even schedule outdoor field trips such as stand up paddle boarding, golf, happy hours, and dinner clubs. Our clients are now friends. This social community is key to feeling accountability to show up to your workout training sessions.

FITNESS AND HEALTH

Did you know you can be fit but still be unhealthy? In my podcast episodes with Dr. Phil Maffetone, we discuss the difference between fitness and health. A few key points:

- Fitness and health can be defined separately: fitness describes the ability to perform a given exercise task and health explains a person's state of well-being, where physiological systems work in harmony.
- Too many athletes are fit but unhealthy.
- Excess high training intensity or training volume and/or excess consumption of processed/refined dietary carbohydrates can contribute to reduced health in athletes and even impair performance.

Our goal here is to get MORE results from your workout sessions in less time without burning out, overtraining, and creating injuries. In other words, we will achieve fitness *and* health. We will do this by avoiding the overtraining spiral where you spend too much time in the black hole above aerobic ceiling heart rate. While the endurance engine is important, so is scheduling days for strength training (the hormonal effect is huge) as well as mobility/flexibility and movement training.

Another important strategy is to watch your type A drive to do all your training sessions by working out two to three times per day. Trust me, this will burn out and break down your body. If you read my book, *Life is Not a Race*, you will learn from my experience that trying to fit every type of workout into an already packed work schedule leads to crash and burn. I don't want you to experience the breakdown of the body systems like I did. Let's find the right amount and type of exercise for your body to promote optimal health and reach your peak performance.

In this course, you will learn how to create a weekly, monthly, and quarterly workout plan routines that offer more focus on lower heart rate training, days outside in nature, strength training and active recovery session days. You will learn how to become Fit *and* Healthy.

Being in nature is so important that I want to expand on this a bit. As a culture, we spend far too much time indoors under fluorescent lights and LED lights. Research shows that being in nature reduces stress and is important for vitamin D levels as well as brain and whole body health. Vitamin D allows one to more effectively use calcium, improves the immune system, helps prevents cancer, and is important for brain function. And no vitamin D conversation is complete without mentioning sunscreen. If your outdoor exercise is early in the morning or in the evening, consider foregoing the sunscreen as it blocks the absorption of Vitamin D. If that does not fit you, remember that only 10-15 minutes of sun exposure daily (without sunscreen) provides adequate levels of vitamin D. Also, while you are at it, take off those sunglasses for a few minutes. According to Dr. Phil Maffetone, the human eye contains photosensitive cells in its retina, with connections directly to the pituitary gland in the brain. Stimulation of these important cells comes from sunlight, in particular, the blue unseen spectrum. A study by Dr. Turner and Dr. Mainster of the University of Kansas School of Medicine, published in the British Journal of Ophthalmology in 2008 states, "these photoreceptors play a vital role in human physiology and health." The effects are not only in the brain, but the whole body.

USING HEART RATE VARIABILITY TO GUIDE WORKOUTS

In order to be Fit *and* Healthy, we must accept that more is not better. Most athletes know getting enough rest after exercise is essential to high-level performance, but many still overtrain and feel guilty when they take a day off. The body repairs and strengthens itself in the time between workouts. Continuous training can actually weaken the strongest athletes. In competitive sports, improved performance is achieved by alternating periods of intensive training with periods of relative rest. Rest is physically necessary so the muscles can repair, rebuild, and strengthen. For recreational athletes, building in rest days can help maintain a better balance between home, work, and fitness goals.

While standardized training programs produce well-documented results, they do not take individual responses into account. Age, gender, race, baseline fitness level and genetic factors are known determinants of individual responses to endurance training.

It turns out that the nervous system becomes "fatigued" when you overtrain. Heart Rate Variability (HRV) is a view of the nervous system and can be used to guide an optimal training program. What exactly is Heart Rate Variability? HRV is the natural variation in time between each heartbeat. If your heart beats at 60 beats/minute it does not beat at 1-second intervals like a metronome; it actually beats at something like .85 seconds, .93 seconds, .98 seconds, 1.2 seconds, etc. which averages out to 1-second intervals or 60 beats/minute.

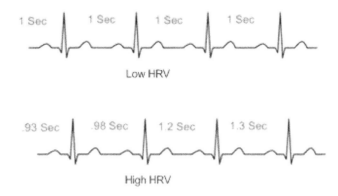

This variation is due to the "push and pull" of the autonomic nervous system. The Autonomic Nervous System (which takes care of things like digestion, breathing, hormone regulation, etc.) has two branches, the Sympathetic and Parasympathetic. The Sympathetic or "Fight or Flight" branch speeds the heart up while the Parasympathetic or "Rest and Repair" branch slows the heart down. These two branches work together to keep the body in equilibrium, and you go through your day.

By measuring your HRV every morning, you can see when you are fatigued and ready for a low exertion or rest day or whether you are recovered and in shape to push it hard. I use SweetBeatHRV's "HRV for Training" feature every day to customize my training. Research shows that by including HRV into your regime, you have better outcomes in the long run by resting when your body is in recovery mode. And don't we all want better outcomes in the long run?

I also use MYZONE heart rate monitor to manage intensity levels. If we want to improve fat burning, optimize our health, and continue to improve performance in daily life and sports, we need to look at our training schedule and have a proper recovery time after a workout.

To lose those last five pounds, gain optimal health benefits, or attain specific sports performance goals, you need to not only avoid training in the black hole, but also by measuring HRV and allowing for recovery days. By training appropriately, as a WHOLEISTIC Athlete, you will start seeing the results you have been trying to achieve for months, stop hanging out on the treadmill or elliptical and learn how to work out efficiently.

HEART RATE TRAINING

How many times does someone start a beginning of a bike or run up a small hill without watching their heart rate? Their heart rate soars up above their anaerobic threshold zone and continues the rest of their workout or endurance race using carbohydrates as their main fuel source. Result? Bonking early in training workout or race and then overeating sugar performance gels or bars to find the energy needed and then battling stomach/GI issues induced by all the sugar-laden supplements. I recommend training by Dr. Maffetone's MAF heart rate formula (180-age) if you can't get a metabolic exercise assessment and if you want to burn fat as your main fuel source and improve your performance in sports.

I have done many podcast interviews with my triathlon coach and the famous athlete, Mark Allen, talking to him about his approach to heart rate training. Many will know Mark as one of the premier American triathletes of all time who is now a coach to high-level triathletes and runs his own coaching business at http://www.markallencoaching.com. He is a partner in another business to promote mental health, stress management, and fitness on all levels called Fit Soul, Fit Body (http://www.fitsoul-fitbody.com/). He is also the co-author of *The Art of Competition* with Nick Borelli. (http://art-of-competition.com/the-book/).

Mark talked about the importance both of heart rate training, and in making certain you are going *slow* enough to build aerobic strength. Aerobic strength is what allows you to endure, and a good aerobic base is essential for being able to stay strong throughout a long race, and throughout the season.

Both Mark and I recognize that trying to focus on aerobic strength and making sure that your heart rate will stay low throughout a training session can be frustrating. We are naturally focused on going harder and faster, and it will take a change in our mindset to spend our time on lower-intensity, aerobic work instead. However, though it may cause some irritation when we force ourselves to go slower and build aerobic strength, the rewards are well worth it, as we can stay strong through a race or throughout the season.

Heart rate training and aerobic exercise also train the body to burn fat instead of calories from carbohydrates. This means that an athlete can tap into a far larger source of energy, and as I pointed out, can free them from the need to be constantly providing the body with more nutrients throughout a race. Aerobic strength is one of the keys to becoming a fat burning machine.

In Mark's coaching program, as I do with my clients, use the MAFF heart rate formula developed by Dr. Phil Maffetone if you don't have access to a metabolic efficiency testing cart.

We have interviewed Dr. Maffetone many times on FIT FAT FAST, and *The WHOLE Athlete* podcast (find in our archives on www.thewholeathletepodcast.com) explained the history of how he came up with the Maffetone formula.

MAF 180 HEART RATE TRAINING

Determine your MAX AEROBIC FUNCTION Heart Rate to improve your performance in endurance sports and improve the ability to burn fat –and many more benefits. (https://philmaffetone.com/180-formula)

The 180 Heart Rate Formula was developed by Dr. Philip Maffetone who went on to coach triathlon greats Mark Allen and Mike Pigg. Even though this formula is over twenty years old, it still seems to be a great starting point especially if you can't get a Metabolic Efficiency Assessment conducted. Train below your MAF heart rate up to ten beats below for your aerobic training zone. Test yourself monthly. Once you stop getting faster, then add one tempo or speed workout per week (talk to your coach).

How did Dr. Maffetone come up with the formula?

The MAF Method looks at critical changes in substrate utilization to define low-intensity exercise in opposition to high-intensity exercise:

Low-intensity exercise is associated with high fat-burning (called Fatmax), and high-intensity exercise is associated with reduced fat-burning and high sugar-burning. Some authors also use Fatmax as a threshold measure for exercise prescription, often referring to it as anaerobic threshold (AerT).

Because of the correspondence of heart rate to markers of substrate utilization and other metabolic activity, the MAF Method identifies the Maximum Aerobic Function Heart Rate (MAF HR) as the heart rate which corresponds with AerT and Fatmax. As we shall see, AerT, Fatmax, and consequently the MAF HR, indicate where the body is most advantageously positioned to:

- *Reap health benefits from exercise.*

- *Develop the aerobic system to increase work rate (running speed, cycling power, etc.) and performance.*
- *Improve the physiological systems necessary to recover from the exercise of all intensities.*

See the rest of the article at:

http://tinyurl.com/MaffetoneWhitePaper

The overwhelming majority of exercise should occur at a low intensity to keep the body healthy, build the aerobic system and improve fat-burning. Modern humans are physiologically better adapted to exercise intensities similar to ones their hominid ancestors evolved with rather than those supported by modern societies. These would have included daily bouts of prolonged, low-intensity, aerobic-based activities, which are primarily fueled by the body's long-term energy source: fats. Lower-intensity exercise has been described as regenerative since it activates and develops the organs, systems, and processes that together exhibit a series of interrelated functions.

These include:
- *Endurance exercise capabilities.*
- *Protection from metabolic syndrome.*
- *Recovery from the high-intensity activity.*
- *Resilience to oxidative stress (aging).*

All these abilities stem from the body's ability to draw reliably and continuously from an abundant fuel source (fats) and a near-limitless supply of reactant (oxygen). A high level of fat-burning bolsters the metabolism and creates positive health outcomes due to its epigenetic effects on gene expression.

The 180 Formula

To find the maximum aerobic heart rate:

1. Subtract your age from 180 (180 – age).

2. Modify this number by selecting a category below that best matches your health profile:
   a. If you have or are recovering from a major illness (heart disease, high blood pressure, an operation or hospital stay, etc.) or you are taking medication, subtract additional ten beats.
   b. If you have not exercised before or have been training inconsistently or injured, have not recently progressed in training or competition, or if you get more than

two colds or bouts of flu per year, or have allergies, subtract an additional five beats.

3. If you've been exercising regularly (at least four times weekly) for up to two years without any of the problems listed in a or b, keep the number (180 – age) the same.

4. If you have been competing for more than two years' duration without any of the problems listed above, and have improved in competition without injury, add five.

For example, if you are forty years old and fit into category b:

180 – 40 = 140, then 140 – 5 = 135 beats per minute.

During your aerobic (Zone 2) training, your heart rate training ranges are set ten beats below the maximum MAF aerobic heart rate. As in the example above, train all your workouts between 125 and 135 beats per minute with the goal of staying as close to 135 as possible (even on hills).

To develop the most efficient aerobic engine, all training should be at or below this level during base building. As the aerobic system develops, you will be able to exercise (bike or run) faster at the same maximum aerobic heart rate. You will have to work harder to get to the MAF heart as 135 BPM in the example above. Once a great aerobic base is developed, an athlete can develop anaerobic function, if needed, depending on race goals and health status.

One major benefit to note of applying the 180 Formula is the biochemical response: production of free radicals is minimal at this training level compared to training at higher heart rates. During exercise, free radicals contribute to degenerative problems, inflammation, heart disease, cancer, and rapid aging.

The MAF Test was developed to track the improvement of the aerobic system across time (see Table 3). For a runner, this test may consist of a three to five mile run on a 400-meter track, while recording the time per mile (or kilometer). For you to do this, decide upon a fixed route or go to a track and choose a distance. Warm up for fifteen minutes then run this predefined route or distance at your MAF heart rate, timing the run. For me, I measure how long it takes to run one mile at a heart rate of 135 BPM. You will need to be able to duplicate the test each month with the exact conditions and time of day.

Increasing speed at the same sub max HR translates to improvement in aerobic function, fat-burning, and can predict faster race performances. It has also been long known that aerobic contribution to energy during maximal exercise such as competition is significant, and increases with the duration of the event.

Read more about the monthly MAF test and start adding into your monthly program. Learn more about Dr. Maffetone's formula, blog, and books at http://philmaffetone.com. You will be amazed by how much you improve over time if you are strict with training at your MAF heart rate. I contribute my excellent aerobic engine to this type of training. Once upon a time, I could do the Boston Marathon in 3:12 and Ironman Canada bike split at 5:12 then run a 3:45 run split to finish a 10:24 Ironman time with a smile on my face and feeling comfortable in the aerobic fat burning zone. You may not have this as a goal; whatever your goals are, you will achieve them if you stick to this method

TRAINING EXAMPLES

What is my weekly routine?

Well, I still train as if I am doing a triathlon by swimming, biking, and running each week (I enjoy it) and I also add two to three strength training workouts. In one of the strength workouts, I make sure I try to lift heavier weights with cardio blasts and then do one workout session per week that focuses on more mobility, stability, and core work. My third strength workout is usually a circuit style with supersets (two exercises back-to-back working for similar muscle groups). I enjoy variety each week so my workouts are never the same. The timer may be used for my intervals instead of counting repetitions, as well as speed changes when lifting weights from super slow to faster-controlled pace.

If I don't have time to go to Yoga or Pilates, I add yoga and Pilates type of movements to my workout sessions. This eliminates the stress I put on myself when I try to fit in two to four more hours of workouts per week (though I love going to my yoga studio and I love doing Pilates Reformer). However, I can't do everything unless I give up something else so I combine them and get some of the benefits of going to a full class.

We must remember the rest of our lives we have to live. Who has time to work out that much plus work full time, run a business (work or family) and have relationships? If you haven't figured it out already too much exercise on top of a busy life workload is another source of stress on your body.

Exercise Suggestions

- Schedule workouts in advance each in your workout log. Keep a daily log of updated completed workouts and energy levels to track progress.

- Meet with a trainer or friend to be accountable.
- Start each morning with easy thirty minutes of low-intensity exercise bike, nature walk, and jog, Pilates, or Yoga. (Zone 1-2 heart rate) in a fasted state (eat breakfast after easy workout).
- If not a beginner, add two to three interval training workouts per week to increase lean body mass improve metabolism and speed up fat loss.
- Our goal is to train your body to utilize fat as the main fuel source and to increase metabolism (strength and interval training – anabolic).
- Get a metabolic resting and exercise test to determine your metabolic profile. Get tested at: https://secure.metabolictypingonline.com
- Listen to your body. Go for a walk instead if you need more recovery. Your body will tell you if you listen.
- Do more mobility, stability, and yoga training. If you can't move right, then you are probably doing more damage than good. Improve your joint mobility and flexibility with a daily practice; five minutes even helps.

Let's look at Primal Endurance training

Brad Kearns, author of the *Primal Endurance* book, shares similar philosophies of training based on his years of experience as an athlete, coach, and individual living life.

The Primal Endurance program advisors say they emphasize the development of the aerobic system and making the human body a fat-burning beast instead of utilizing carbohydrates, thereby escaping dependence on the carbohydrates. Many people eat a lot of sugar and then they force themselves to do a strenuous exercise which can eventually lead to oxidative damage to the cells accelerated aging. Doing excessive and physically exhausting exercise is never recommended. Recent research shows that human genes, hormones and other chemicals in the human body respond very well even by doing low-level movements. This provides the benefits without putting one in a state of stress. On the other end of the spectrum, many people work at a desk all day and do not move very much for eight hours. This too is unhealthy.

While the ideal is to stay in the middle of both extremes, the question arises "how can it be done?" Stressful exercises lead to the production of fight and flight hormones which are never beneficial. These hormones keep a person in a hyperactive state even in a normal environment. This is one reason to build a proper aerobic pace and to become good at burning fats which are the essence of success.

People should slowly get ready for any endurance sport by keeping their pace within aerobic pace limits so that, day after day, they can build without any interruption from the physically exhaustive workouts. That said, shorter duration high-intensity bursts do not keep a person's stress hormonal level in the blood long enough to create a problem. These kinds of brief stressful events are much more nurturing to a person's body and health; like a twenty-minute workout can give you an incredible fitness boost. High-intensity training for a brief period of time is more beneficial than over stressful training. This includes brief occasions of high-intensity maximum effort sprinting and strength training.

Now a question arises: how often should you include these high-intensity exercises? It depends on the time (in days, months, years) dedicated to just aerobically paced exercise and the nature of competition for which one is getting ready for. Sometimes it can take one or two years before you include high-intensity training. Some people are so damaged by excessive or chronic exhaustive workouts that they'll take longer to be ready. Gentle pace aerobic training is a key to getting ready for a big event.

It's also recommended to do periodization. This is where people focus on aerobically-paced training for some defined period of time and add periods of intensity via strength training exercises. Proper endurance athletes often spend fifteen minutes of every training hour doing flexibility and mobility work like running drills, high knees, butt kicks, etc.

And last, but not the least, the nutritional needs of an athlete are extreme as compared to the general population so eating nutritional calories is mandatory for peak performance.

My Primal Blueprint and Primal Endurance podcast host, author, and athlete, Brad Kearns shares his workout tips:

For the past ten years, I have modified my fitness regimen away from narrow endurance focus (including the extremely health-destructive chronic cardio training regimen that I followed for fifteen years as a college runner and then pro triathlete) to a more balanced regimen featuring comfortable aerobic workouts (i.e., jogging slowly every morning with dogs), regular brief, intense strength training sessions, and occasional all-out sprints:

Brad's fitness routine:
1. Daily very comfortable jogging (HR 130 BPM max) of thirty minutes with dogs
2. Brief strength training sessions lasting from eight to twelve minutes, one to three days/week. Extremely high-intensity full-body exercises (heavy bar and cable stuff in gym, or stretch cords and decline Spiderman pushups in backyard)
3. Occasional all-out sprints: three times per month and usually just six times per

hundred meters on grass, along with ten minutes of quite challenging technique drills.

4. Five minutes of technique drills interspersed into daily runs so I can handle sprinting

Main goals: Speed golf competition requiring great aerobic endurance and High jump competition requiring explosive power. The training regimen fuels these goals without compromising my health.

MOVING THROUGHOUT THE DAY

An important topic that is finally getting attention is that most people spend too much time sitting and not getting enough movement throughout the day. Even fit athletes who work out regularly can be compromising their health by sitting too much. The typical workout at the gym is time spent on the cardio machines (often sitting on a bike) and maybe some high rep strength training routine on the machine circuit. Many of these machines involve sitting for a long time.

Then what do most people do the rest of the day after their workout? They sit. Research indicates that temporary vigorous exercise does not compensate for the damage incurred by prolonged sitting and that the minimum number of times you need to stand from sitting is at least 35 times per day. This counteracts the cardiovascular health risks that sitting enables.

An article in USA Today reported, *"The risk of heart failure was more than double for men who sat for at least five hours a day outside of work and didn't exercise very much compared with men who were physically active and sat for less than two hours a day... The risk was lowest for men who exercised the most and sat for fewer than two hours a day...*

Government statistics show almost half of people report sitting more than six hours a day, and 65 percent say they spend more than two hours a day watching TV. 'If you've been sitting for an hour, you've been sitting too long,' says James Levine, co-director of Obesity Solutions at Mayo Clinic in Phoenix and Arizona State University".

This study, which followed 82,000 men over ten years, also confirms that a regular fitness routine does not reduce the effects of prolonged sitting.

So what can you do? Move your body frequently throughout the day. It turns out that the act of standing from a seated position has positive cardiovascular effects. Specifically:

- Set a timer or use your activity tracker such as a Fitbit or ZoomHRV to remind you to stand every 15 minutes
- Get an adjustable standing desk and better yet get a treadmill desk
- When you are on the phone, get up and walk around
- Park far away – less time sitting, more time walking
- Take the stairs – it will take longer so less sitting time

METABOLICALLY EFFICIENCY

Do you burn sugar or fat for your main fuel source? Do you fuel your fire with quick burning kindling or slow burning logs?

How efficient is your body at utilizing stores of carbohydrate and fat at various training heart rates, duration and at rest?

As we discussed in the previous chapter, we should be burning fat while we are sitting, sleeping, driving our cars, working, etc. The challenge is that most people have a diet and stress levels that make sugar burners. In addition, many do high of heart rate training at day after day. We can learn how to become a fat burning machine by teaching our bodies how to depend on fat for its main fuel source while preserving our carbohydrates stores which is what the term being "metabolically efficient" is about.

The way we train and what we eat makes a difference in our ability to use stored fat for fuel as well as stress and sleep of course:

- Do you train and compete in endurance events two hours or longer?
- Do you eat a high carb meal before your workout?
- Do you eat 200-300 calories per hour of sports drinks, gels, and bars when you train or race?
- Do you ever have GI distress or problems?
- Do you feel tired after eating and exercising?
- Are you trying to lose weight and perform better?

I have been training for endurance events since I was twenty-five years old, including long-distance cycling events, Ironman distance triathlons, marathons to 50K trail races. For the last fifteen plus years, I have wondered why I kept eating a high carb healthy meal before a workout, then ate gels, bars, and drink mixes to keep me fueled during my workout. I have raced with various drink mixes and still have a habit of eliminating excess liquid from my bloated belly while I am racing (typically on the bike).

Eating a high carb typical athlete food plan never made sense to me. For years, I have trained by heart rate, built up my aerobic engine, and improved my ability to burn fat for fuel. Now, I have finally figured out how to not only train right, but eat right, to be metabolically efficient.

As a coach and trainer, I have trained clients for years on how to train by heart rate and conducted metabolic assessments with New Leaf Metabolic Assessments on the treadmill and/or bikes. The information from the metabolic assessments is invaluable for any endurance athlete training for an event or anyone just trying to lose fat weight

We can now also figure out how to improve and move your Metabolic Efficiency Point through a proper training and nutrition program. We need to figure out which heart rates do we burn the most fat for fuel for endurance training, tempo ranges and speed work, but also what to eat (or not eat) before, during and after workouts.

Definition of Metabolic Efficiency: The body's ability to utilize fat as the main fuel source while sparing the limited amounts of stored carbohydrates. Which fuel source makes more sense to use for endurance events?

A metabolic assessment will determine and measure the following information:
- Aerobic Base (AB): the highest heart rate (and range) where you burn the highest percentage of fat for fuel
- Anaerobic Threshold (AT): where you are no longer burning fat for fuel; VCO_2 is higher than VO_2.
- Respiratory Exchange Ratio (RER or RQ value)
- Metabolic Efficiency Point (MEP): where you begin to burn more carbohydrates than fat
- Peak volume of Oxygen (VO_2 ml/kg/min)
- Recovery heart rate and fuel source used post-AT

Training Zones/RER:
Zone 1: Recovery and Warm-up
Zone 2: Endurance training
Zone 3: Tempo

Zone 4: Threshold

Zone 5: VO2 training intervals

Why should you train below your MEP or AT?

Once you go near or above your tested anaerobic threshold, you are no longer burning fat for fuel or depending on carbohydrates for fuel. If you continue to train or race above your AT, you are limited to fuel source (carbohydrates = 1,200 calories as stored muscle glycogen), and you will need to consume more calories each hour to resupply your muscle glycogen stores. If you want to tap into the estimated 80,000 calories of stored energy from the fat fuel, then you need to stay in your aerobic ranges the ENTIRE time of your workout or at least the majority first half or more.

From the Metabolic Assessment, we can measure your recovery heart rate and fuel uses (RER) after you hit your anaerobic threshold (you are not using fat for fuel anymore). Even if your heart rate drops back to zone two aerobic endurance training or zone one recovery range, you may still be burning primarily carbohydrates for fuel. Yes, the assessment can tell if you return to burning a similar percent of fat calories at lower heart rates post anaerobic heart rates, and this is your goal.

"BLACK HOLE" TRAINING VERSES MAF

There is another heart rate range known as the Black Hole training area. What is the black hole training style? Technically, the Black Hole is a very narrow heart-rate zone from 100 to 105 percent of your aerobic threshold (AT). Non-technically, the Black Hole is when you start running just fast enough to where it becomes difficult to carry on a conversation (known as the "Talk Test"). These are junk miles when you perform all your training sessions at one heart rate range. It's not easy, yet not too hard. You feel like you had a hard workout, but not too exhausting like doing all-out sprints. Often people train in the black hole three to five times a week for the typical forty-five to sixty-minute workout set on the same machine or on the same course. This same old routine probably does not elicit any significant training responses. It's Groundhog Day for endurance training.

Ben Greenfield talks a lot about the Black Hole training in his book, podcast, and blogs: http://tinyurl.com/GreenfieldEndurance.

So, how do we train to avoid being stuck in Groundhog Day doing the same workout at the same intensity on the same course every day? Once you have built up your aerobic base and your foundation, then you can try adding one or two short high-intensity workouts in per week. That is, after months of strictly training at or below your metabolic efficiency tested or MAF predicted aerobic training range. When you have passed the test, and are ready to graduate, try the 80/20 training for endurance athletes. Here is an interesting research study: http://www.sportsci.org/2009/ss.htm.

The 80:20 Rule for Intensity

- There is reasonable evidence that an 80:20 ratio of low to high-intensity training (HIT) gives excellent long-term results among endurance athletes training daily.

- Low intensity (typically below 2 mM blood lactate), longer duration training is effective in stimulating physiological adaptations and should not be viewed as wasted training time.

- Over a broad range, increases in total training volume correlate well with improvements in physiological variables and performance.

- HIT should be a part of the training program of all those who exercise and endurance athletes. However, about two training sessions per week using this modality seems to be sufficient for achieving performance gains without inducing excessive stress.

- The effects of HIT on physiology and performance are fairly rapid, but rapid plateau effects are seen as well. To avoid premature stagnation and ensure long-term development, training volume should increase systematically.

- When already well-trained athletes markedly intensify training with more HIT over twelve to forty-five weeks, the impact is equivocal.

- In athletes with an established endurance base and tolerance for relatively high training loads, intensification of training may yield small performance gains at acceptable risk.

- An established endurance base built from reasonably high volumes of training may be an important precondition for tolerating and responding well to a substantial increase in training intensity over the short term.

- Periodization of training by elite athletes is achieved with reductions in total volume, and a modest increase in the volume of training performed above the lactate threshold. An overall polarization of training intensity characterizes the transition from preparation to competition mesocycles. The basic intensity distribution remains similar throughout the year.

If you are not an endurance athlete training for a long-distance race and just want to be healthy and lose weight, then how should you train? As we have discussed on many podcasts, doing high-intensity interval training (HIIT) is beneficial to improve post-workout metabolism, but again, more is not better. Less is better. I tell my clients to have a purpose to each workout as well as focusing on following through with your game plan to achieve specific goals, not garbage miles.

Another mentor over the years who first taught me about training with a heart rate monitor is a longtime friend, Sally Edwards of Heart Zones USA training systems. Sally is the originator of heart rate training, and she literally wrote the book on it, called _The Heart Rate Monitor Book_ back in 1993. She was the first athlete to recognize the value of heart rate monitors and keeping track of where your heart rate is when you are training.

I talked to Sally about the training regimes that emphasize HIIT too much. The result is that people are enjoying workouts less and doing it from high intensity to burnout.

The common feature of these approaches is the lack of recovery time. In fact, the pendulum has swung too far to one end of the spectrum. While it was once common to train exclusively for endurance, for very long periods with minimal intensity using the MAFF formula now many people train almost exclusively in the red zone by doing short and intense high-intensity interval workouts. One extreme or the other is not ideal, and the body responds better to variability. Sally describes as variation training.

As with our nutrition plan, the body responds better to changing things up. The result is doing too much high intensity will either exhaust people or leave them working out in moderate intensity. This happens because they are unwilling to let themselves recover. What is helpful to alleviate this is variation between different heart rate zones. The MYZONE training zones are slightly different (five different zones where you also earn points—My Effort Points (MEPs), but the same principles—train in the appropriate zones based on fitness goals, and to allow sufficient recovery time in between workout sessions.

Sally Edward's heart rate zone program identifies three zones to keep heart rate training simple:

1. Blue or least intense zone; recovery area (blue tile for MYZONE 60-70% max heart rate)
2. Yellow or moderate intensity zone; aerobic; (blue to green tile for MYZONE 70-80% heart rate)

3. Red, which is high intensity; anaerobic. (yellow and red tiles for MYZONE 80-90% for yellow zone then red zone is 90-100% max heart rate)

No zone (or grey zone for MYZONE) is a goal in and of itself. Train hard and recover harder. We should be training in recovery zones the day after a high-intensity interval training zone day. Each zone has advantages and you're only able to effectively utilize those advantages if you make your workouts variable. Check it out at www.heartzones.com and http://thesallyedwardscompany.com/

In my studio, we started implementing the MYZONE heart rate training program so client's effort levels can be visible on the big screen television. The MYZONE heart rate belt can be purchased online (use facility code **FITFORUS001** for a discount) and worn by clients for their personal training sessions or group training sessions. Now, we can see their heart rate on the big screen television and their colored tiled zone is visible on the screen or big board.

As a trainer and a coach, I have been waiting for almost twenty years to have this type of technology available to us in a fitness studio or gym. After many years teaching spin class by heart rate and pace with half the clients pushing the pace and the others just enjoying the social environment, now we have visible evidence of each client's effort level.

We can design workouts for each individual client that will keep their heart rate when appropriate in their recovery (blue zone), aerobic (green zone), tempo (yellow) or anaerobic (red).

My clients can keep their heart rate aerobic during strength training exercises as we can now experiment with strength movements and visibly see what happens to the heart rate or effort level when they sit or lie down as compared to a total body functional strength movement.

I focus on functional strength training movements for clients for life movement patterns as well as sports specific so we don't use the machine circuit that you see people resting over in the big box gyms and completely losing their posture and alignment. A total body movement or a functional strength movement pattern would be integrating the entire body instead of a single muscle group exercise.

For example, instead of sitting on the Lat Pull machine, we now stand in a lunge position or a squat while we pull the bar to our chest. We often stand on one leg or an off-set squat position when doing upper body movements or a standing chest press on the cable machine. I usually do single arm and leg movements in combination with another movement. Also, we don't do all our core exercises on the mat. We do more standing on the cables or with tubing.

Now, combine the total body movements with a heart rate monitor. We can measure the effort level required by the client with the MYZONE effort level points program (MEPS). This provides a more time efficient workout for the client as well as metabolically efficient as we can add more cardio blasts or HIIT (high-intensity interval training) sets into the workout to drive metabolism up post workout (EPOC). Get more out of your workouts in less time by combining movements and exercises while wearing your heart rate monitors.

You won't need to do your cardio workout on the machines after your strength training session. You now will do what I call an all in one workout...we can get our cardio, strength, core, mobility, agility, and sport-specific movements in one workout session in thirty minutes.

Next, we can work on programming the ideal workout routine for the week based on the heart rate in the previous workout or the MYZONE workout report. My goal as a trainer and coach is to avoid overtraining my client by only training in the yellow and red tiles or zones every two to three days. We should not train in red zone back to back days. We need recovery time in between hard high-intensity workouts. While the best way to determine recovery is by using SweetBeatHRV's HRV for Training feature, not all of my clients have the discipline to do this so I go with the generic recovery schedule.

In general, if a client does a HITT type of workout, the following day they need to do a low-intensity recovery workout and stay in the green or blue tile or zone. If we rotate hard workouts, then we are rested and ready to go hard on the specific scheduled day instead of being fatigued and exhausted every day. We need to work hard but recover harder. Once again I highly recommend using HRV to determine individual recovery status.

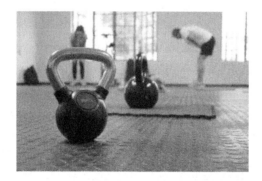

Try using MYZONE into your workouts and use our *FITFORUS001 facility code* to join our community. See the MYZONE app on your phone or log in to your account on their website. Order your monitor and get started this week on changing or improving how you train or how your trainer trains you.

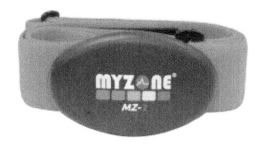

MYZONE® Benefits:

- See your calories, heart rate, and effort in real-time with easy-to-follow colors
- Automatic email feedback on all your exercise motivates you to stay on track
- View your training efforts via a personalized free app and online account
- Measuring effort levels the playing field and enables competition against yourself or friends
- Monitor your food intake through the free app
- Stay accountable to your health targets with our simple goal setting
- Connect with friends and motivate progress through a personalized social feed
- Participate in challenges with friends and other users all over the world
- Earn rewards through status rankings linked to attaining world health guidelines
- Benefit from accurate calorie burn feedback during all your exercise routines
- Gain exclusive access to zone match classes
- Make exercise fun

Speaking of making exercise fun, I did a podcast with a fellow fitness professional, Jonathan Ross, on FUN-TENSITY. He has the right idea in that we need to create workout plans that are fun and make your brain work. The result is laughter and smiles while you don't even realize you are exercising as well as keeping your mind focused on the moment and being present. Jonathan is on a mission to teach others—coaches and clients—how to play.

One of Jonathan's favorite quotes that captures this idea is from Stuart Brown's book, *Play:*

"The opposite of play is not work... the opposite of play is depression." Play and work are mutually supportive; neither can thrive without the other. We need the newness of play, its sense of flow, and being in the moment. We need a sense of discovery and liveliness that it provides. We also need the purpose of work, the sense we are doing service for others, and more

of us need to feel competent.

He teaches people to "lose you in play to find yourself in fitness. If you are lost in play, it frees you from a focus on the intensity of the experience."

Source: Jonathan Ross, http://www.aionfitness.com/

Before wrapping up the discussion on exercise—which I could write on for several books—let me share more tips for you.

Invest in a foam roller, BOSU, a TRX, and even a yoga strap or rope. Find mobility exercises to do with your bodyweight alone and with the above mobility toys for opening your spine, shoulders, chest, hips, and more. Find tips on my Pinterest board: https://www.pinterest.com/WholesticMethod/

We talked a lot in this chapter about heart rate training and metabolic efficiency, but I want to make sure you understand the importance of strength training in your weekly routine to boost your fat burning hormones as well as to feel better and of course look better. Being stronger improves your confidence, self-esteem, body composition, hormones and of course your metabolism. We don't need to be afraid (Listen, ladies...) of lifting heavier weights; we are not going to look like The Incredible Hulk. To improve your hormones, you should lift weights one to three times a week for even five to thirty minutes. Less is more if you create the right workout routine.

Check out my YouTube channel and Instagram for workout ideas you can follow. Links are found at the end of the manual.

I must add the importance of adding strength training for the hormonal effect on the body, as well. You can ask Dr. Google for details on the hormonal effect of strength training. Also, downloads my podcast with Keoni Teta from *Metabolic Effect* and *Primal Endurance* co-author, Brad Kearns. We touch a little on hormones in our other chapters, but again hormones could be an entire book. Don't think females are the only ones with hormones and that we get edgy once a month then hit menopause – then we get really hormonal.

Strength training influences many of our hormones including:

- Testosterone
- Growth Hormones
- Insulin
- Glucagon
- Cortisol

MICHOL DALCOURT

Michol Dalcourt is an expert in human movement and performance. He is the founder of Institute of Motion (IoM) and the inventor of the fitness device called VIPR. He's also a co-founder of PTA global for fitness professionals.

Michol focuses on physical innovation strategies not only for performance, but also for management and sustainability of biological functions. There are some pros and cons of training if the dosage and exposure are too high. We all need a healthy baseline so we can get better results and high performance.

When asked about the meaning of stress, Michol replied, "We all are under stress, including animals. If you put an animal in the cage and provide it with food daily, even then you will see it would be out of balance because it can't move anymore and will be in stress about its food, movement etc. In the same way, we have personal, work-related, and physical stress."

How can a person improve his or her performance?

In response to this point, Michol said movement itself is a stress. It's a mechanical stress which we need because that signals things to happen in our body. So, we do know that lack of movement doesn't facilitate the right signaling pathways. From a movement perspective, we would know that lack of movement and exposure to mechanical stress is going to affect muscles, making them smaller (this is called atrophy). Our blood volume decreases and so we have frail tissues.

WHAT IS MOVEMENT TRAINING, AND WHAT IS ITS IMPACT ON THE SPORTS TRAINING WE DO?

Michol explained we should adopt those exercises suitable to our body and those our body easily accepts. People try to do heavy exercises in the gym all day and they get nothing except body loss and sometimes muscle injuries. Exercises should be variable and sustainable and keep in view four quadrants (see below.) Always try to do variable exercises so your body gets nourished. Sending your children to the farm instead of a gym is better because you only get stress in gym whereas, at the farm, you get different positions as well as exercises.

What precautionary measures should we take to avoid injuries?

In reply to this question, he told us our body cannot do the same task for a long time like someone can dig a ditch whole day because of his body movement, position vary every time but if we do gym exercise repeatedly we will not be able to perform it for a longer period. He is not against the gym exercises, but he suggested other exercises must be a part of our routine.

WHAT ARE FOUR QUADRANTS, AND HOW THEY ARE USED IN TRAINING SESSIONS?

Michol explained all quadrants through examples:

1. Bench-press exercise for the chest, so the first quadrant is loaded and linear strength building exercise for the chest. We put on the load repeatedly and it leads to hypertrophy.

2. The the second quadrant is unloaded linear training consideration that might be a body weight linear part. Push-ups are different from bench-pressing because our body is moving and our hands are static in push-ups and vice versa. Most of life depends on body and motion, in most of the gym exercises our body is static and hands are in a motion and in our life hands are still and body is in motion.

3. The third quadrant is unloaded movement or multi-planer training. Crawling base push-ups is an example of this quadrant.

4. The fourth and last quadrants are loaded multi-planer training. Grabbing cable at your shoulder side and so all the body parts like our hands, body, and feet all have different positions at every step.

So, these are four exercises—a Bench-Press, a Push-ups, a Crawling Push-ups, and a standing cable press—that are all chest-based, they are all pushing and strength based, but there is a high degree of variability and we should do all of them to improve our health. Learn more at https://instituteofmotion.com.

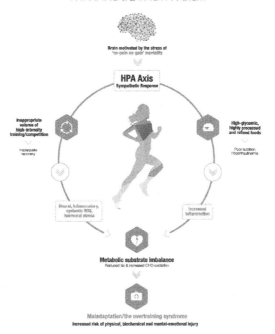

FINAL THOUGHTS

A note to my fellow endurance athlete friends: we are typically Type-A competitive athletes. We may struggle to stick with the MAF training heart rate ranges especially when other people pass you or if you train with workout friends. Try doing most of your workouts solo or stay in the back. If you want to avoid burnout and breakdown in the body, you should try committing to training at or below your aerobic training ranges as set by a metabolic test or with Dr. Maffetone's formula. Make sure you pace yourself by your heart rate during the exercise session, turn off your pace screen, or power meter numbers to keep you strict on sticking with your heart rate range.

Remember to have a purpose for each workout session, add active recovery days and strength training, as well as measuring your heart rate variability (HRV) daily to test if your body is ready to work out again or if you need to reschedule your training session.

When using the MAF formula for building your aerobic engine and metabolic efficiency, put your ego aside. You may need to spend more workouts training solo so you can pace yourself by your heart rate, not with someone else next to you. Also, be aware of using Strava Segments to set personal records and be the king of the mountain—as well as your power meters—when you are in the aerobic engine training phase.

Ride your own ride... run your own run. Stick to building the aerobic engine until you add intervals. Be strict and make the commitment so you will be rewarded by going faster at low aerobic heart rate, recover faster, improve performance, and decrease the risk of breakdown and burnout.

I had to put my ego away after my bout with chronic stress disease (more about my personal journey in my book, *Life is Not a Race*). Honestly, I was trying to get my endurance and speed back to where it was before my health fell like the domino effect. When it came to swimming and cycling and running, I had to go back to following the plan that always worked for me in the past. This was training by MAF heart rate range and ignoring my pace for now.

I use my MYZONE Heart Rate monitor with my Garmin watch then download (Bluetooth is the best invention) to Garmin and connect then to Strava. This allows me to track and measure my progress, plus it keeps me honest and accountable to all my followers on MYZONE community and Strava.

When I was setting PR times in my races, it was because I trained by heart rate with the MAF aerobic engine ranges that my coach Mark Allen uses in his training programs. I continued to get faster at my lower heart rates. On race day, I was racing with a smile on my face – happy and having fun. That is what happens when you train by your heart and avoid burning out and breaking down your body.

Be patient grasshopper... and you will be rewarded.

Plus, don't you want to be burning fat for fuel and not sugar? If you stay below your tested max aerobic training ranges, you will be burning fat for fuel. So, don't sneak out of your training range because of your training partners or you are going up a hill. Too much time above your aerobic max heart rate range stimulates the stress hormone. We are to only run from a lion a few times... a few bursts so do your aerobic training below your 180-Age number and then add your heavy strength training with some high-intensity bursts.

The big five WHOLESTIC Method Exercise tips for becoming a fat burner:

1. _____
2. _____
3. _____
4. _____
5. _____

The WHOLESTIC Method to improving fat loss, health, and performance for life and sports by working from the inside out.

References: Strength Training & Hormonal Effect

http://www.ncbi.nlm.nih.gov/pubmed/15831061
http://tinyurl.com/WomenStrengthTrng
http://tinyurl.com/InfluencerOfFat
http://tinyurl.com/ResistanceExercise
http://www.bodybuilding.com/fun/draper42.htm
http://www.ncbi.nlm.nih.gov/pubmed/10484567
http://www.ncbi.nlm.nih.gov/pubmed/279

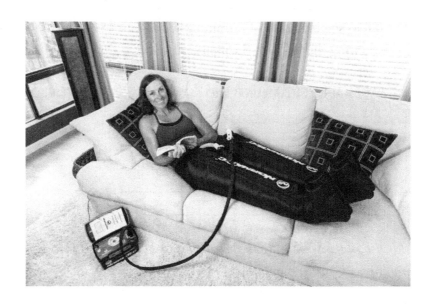

Element #3
SLEEP

Poor quantity and quality of sleep seem to be growing issues in our society. A 2013 Gallup poll reveals that forty percent (40%) of Americans are not getting the recommended seven to nine hours of sleep each night. Excessive use and dependence on our electronic devices like computers, phones, and tablets, as well as checking social media and watching TV late at night can trick our body into thinking it is daytime. Light from these devices stimulates our skin and eyes, brain, and hormonal system to think it is morning and time to wake up.

To make matters worse, it has become trendy and an actual status symbol for some people to not get much sleep. While many people claim, with pride, that they only need four or five hours of sleep each night, only five percent (5%) of the population carries the genetic mutation of the gene DEC2 that allows them to get by on six hours of sleep. According to an article in Scientific America, if normal people (without the mutation) get less than six hours of sleep, "after a few days, you will see some negative impact."

To make matters even worse is the reliance of so many people to sleeping pills. While some people can successfully use sleeping pills for short-term insomnia (like jet lag), many more become dependent on them. The CDC estimates that more than nine million Americans used sleeping pills in 2009. According to the Addiction Center, thirty-eight million prescriptions for Ambien were written between 2006 and 2011.

The Huffington Post wrote, "Although the Ambien prescribing information warned, in small print, that medications in the hypnotic class had occasional side effects including sleep walking, "abnormal thinking," and "strange behavior," these behaviors were listed as extremely rare, and any anecdotal evidence of "sleep driving," "sleep eating," or "sleep shopping"—all behaviors now associated with Ambien blackouts—were characterized as unusual quirks, or attributed to mixing the medication with alcohol. It wasn't until Patrick Kennedy's 2006 middle-of-the-night car accident and subsequent explanation to arriving officers that he was running late for a vote that the bizarre side effects of Ambien began to receive national attention. Kennedy claimed that he had taken the sleep aid and had no recollection of the events that night." So seriously, if you are a regular user of Ambien or other sleep aids, please, please do your homework and get off of them. Seek help from a health professional if needed just do it.

Sleep is absolutely essential for fat loss, health, and performance for life and sports. Unfortunately, most people trade off time sleeping to find more hours in the day to be what they think is productive. Sadly, it is creating the opposite effect.

The long-term effects of sleep deprivation are real. It drains your cognitive abilities and puts your physical health at risk. Your emotional state is compromised making you more prone to mood swings. Because your nervous system and immune system repair and protect your body from the effects of daily living, your immune system may be severely weakened with long-term sleep deprivation. To make matters worse, sleep affects the levels of two weight-related hormones, leptin, and ghrelin, which control feelings of hunger and fullness. A lack of sleep also prompts your body to release higher levels of insulin after you eat, and as we have learned here that is not a good thing. We want stable insulin levels as we turn ourselves into fat burning machines. And that means burning fat while we sleep.

BURNING FAT WHILE WE SLEEP?

Yes, it is true, you should be burning fat while you sleep. However, you probably aren't if you are chronically sleep deprived or are eating the wrong foods before bed. How do our sleep habits relate to how efficient we are at burning fat for fuel at rest (including while we sleep) and during exercise? Lack of sleep and lack of *quality* sleep interferes with cellular rebuilding, recovery, and rejuvenation time. The brain and the body need sleep to repair and prepare us for the next day.

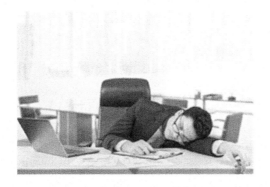

SLEEP AND HORMONES

Many of us have disrupted sleep/wake cycles which interfere with the natural release of "restore and repair" hormones. During our sleep cycle, we have a natural release of melatonin, growth hormones, and other immune-boosting benefits. Our physical repair cycle begins around 10:00 p.m. until 2:00 a.m. and then our psychological repair kicks in between 2:00 a.m. and 6:00 a.m. in his book *How to Eat, Move and be Healthy*, Paul Chek teaches about the importance of sleep as many of our hormones are

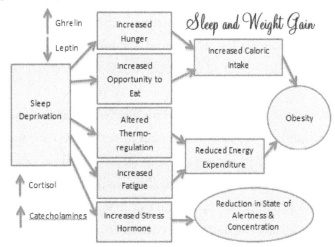

released with the cycle of the sun. According to Paul, we should be winding down and relaxing from sunset until 10:00 p.m. at which time we should go to sleep and start the physical repair phase of our sleep cycle. As mentioned, this is followed by psychogenic repairs at around 2:00 am and continues for the next four hours (if we sleep that long). Most people miss this window as they stay up too late at night and wake up too early in the morning.

The hormones Cortisol and Melatonin play an important role in our overall health and alertness and are intimately tied to our sleep cycle and light exposure. Cortisol, as well as melatonin, has a twenty-four-hour circadian rhythm. In the morning, Cortisol is at its peak around 9:00 a.m. and gradually decreases around noon before it dips down at 3:00-4:00 p.m. when people feel sleepy. There is a continuous drop until midnight when it reaches its minimum value and it starts increasing again and peaks at 9:00 a.m. Cortisol levels increase in response to light and prepare us to tackle the day ahead. However, if we are exposed to artificial light after dark (especially blue light) we training our body that it is time to wake up when it is actually time to go to sleep. Our brain interprets chronic exposure to fluorescent lights, computer screens, and television monitors as morning sunlight. This disrupts the 24-hour Cortisol cycle and can leave us waking groggy and feeling unrested.

The big cortisol surge should happen around 6:00-7:00 a.m. when the brain relays the message to the pituitary glands and then they tell the adrenal glands to execute an order. For many, cortisol production by the adrenal glands surges at 2:00 a.m. This causes people with a broken cortisol cycle to wake up in the middle of the night. Then the stress of "I need to sleep" kicks in, and the brain, via the pituitary, tells the adrenals to make more cortisol.

Remember chronic exposure to anything usually shows up as chronic something in the body. Chronic fatigue, headaches, nagging injuries, depression, and more may be a result of our disrupted sleep cycles and chronic exposure to artificial light, especially after the sun has gone down.

Besides being on a natural 24-hour rhythm, cortisol is one of our stress hormones released by our adrenal glands. Too much cortisol from stress in the evening can keep you from getting a deep sleep, cause you to wake up frequently during the night as well as leave you waking up in the morning feeling exhausted. This can become a vicious cycle. Too much stress, in any form, interrupts the sleep cycle and then our body doesn't have the sleep to time to repair, rebuild, and stabilize the hormones. This can result in the release of more cortisol when you may already have too much in your body from excessive emotional, physical, or environmental stress. I talk about this vicious cycle in my book, *Life is Not a Race*. We often don't sleep well at night due to various reason, then wake up tired, drink too much coffee all day then are wired at night when we are supposed to be mellow and ready to fall asleep.

How do we get more quality sleep? Stay tuned for a few tips to help find a good night's sleep.

SLEEP AND WEIGHT GAIN

Let's get to an important topic... fat loss. What do fat loss and sleep have to do with one another? Well, lack of sleep could be contributing to your weight gain via something called leptin resistance.

A study by S. Taheri *et.al.* titled "Short Sleep Duration is Associated with Reduced Leptin, Elevated Ghrelin, and Increased Body Mass Index" concluded:

> *Participants with short sleep had reduced leptin and elevated ghrelin. These differences in leptin and ghrelin are likely to increase appetite, possibly explaining the increased BMI observed with short sleep duration. In Western societies, where chronic sleep restriction is common and the food is widely available, changes in appetite regulatory hormones with sleep curtailment may contribute to obesity.*

Find more on *Leptin Resistance* in our hormone and gut health chapter, but also watch http://tinyurl.com/YouTubeLeptinResistance

It shouldn't come as a surprise to hear that sleep and sugar consumption are connected - too much sugar in your diet can influence your quality of sleep. Dr. Mercola writes about the lack of sleep and sugar cravings in one of his many blog reports about the hormones leptin (satiety) and ghrelin (hunger) hormones:

> When you're sleep deprived, leptin (the hormone that signals satiety) falls, while ghrelin (which signals hunger) rises. In one 2010 study, three researchers found that people who slept only four hours for two consecutive nights experienced eighteen percent (18%) reduction in leptin and twenty-eight percent (28%) increase in ghrelin.

The combination of reducing leptin (makes you feel full and satisfied) and increasing ghrelin (tells you if you are hungry) will increase your appetite. Combine this increased appetite with the lack of sleep and you may experience increased food cravings.

After your evening meal, any additional eating is usually mindless snacking and is often full of carbs and sugars. We may also feel "snacky" because we didn't eat the right ratio of macronutrients based on our metabolic type which would help us feel full for four hours after our meal (see my website www.thewholesticmethod.com for the Metabolic Typing link). I often tell my clients to follow this rule: The kitchen is closed after dinner.

If you go to bed with high blood sugar levels, you may be waking up in the middle of the night hungry because you are experiencing low blood sugar – another reason to get off the blood sugar roller coaster and change your eating habits. You will sleep better if you eat the right foods for you. Listen to your body and take a step back when you find yourself mindlessly grabbing snacks after dinner or before bedtime.

Dr. Mercola also talks about the sugar cravings experienced by a sugar burning metabolism.

> As mentioned, getting too little sleep also dramatically decreases the sensitivity of your insulin receptors, which will raise your insulin levels. This, too, is a surefire way to gain weight, as the insulin will seriously impair your body's ability to burn and digest fat. It also increases your risk of diabetes. In short, sleep deprivation puts your body in a pre-diabetic state, which can lead to increased weight and decreased health.

SUGAR AND SLEEP

As I continue my research and education on the impact on sleep on our health for fat loss, health, and performance, I learned how important it is to balance our blood sugar levels. I started testing my own blood sugar levels in the morning, after meals and workouts for my own education. I can tell when I ate too much sugar (fruit for me), but now I can test that I spiked my blood sugar levels up for hours after I ate a meal with too many carbs for my body.

Everyone is different, but I strongly suggest testing your own blood sugar levels to discover what you should be eating especially in the evening before bed so you don't go to sleep on the blood sugar roller coaster. Once our blood sugar levels increase—hyperglycemia—we have a crash a few hours later with low blood sugar after our fat storing hormone insulin was released to help lower our blood sugar levels. What happens when our blood sugar levels drop down too low? Well, then we are hungry and need to eat again and get on what I always call the Blood Sugar Roller Coaster Ride.

The hormone insulin moves the excess sugar in the bloodstream into the liver and muscles (glycogen energy storage), but when we are already full the sugar is moved into fat cells for storage (body fat). Hopefully, you can appreciate why eating in the evening right before bedtime puts you at risk of disrupting your sleep cycle.

Think about it this way:

Sugar turns to fat.
Eat sugar and gain weight.
Eat fat and lose fat.

I had T-shirts made for my sugar detox clients with this quote on the back. We should be burning fat when we are performing low heart rate activities and at rest, including sleeping for seven to nine hours per night.

HOW DOES GETTING STUCK IN THE BLOOD SUGAR ROLLER COASTER IMPACT OUR SLEEP CYCLE?

If you eat carbs before bed and spike your blood sugar levels, you risk waking up in the middle of the night with a low blood sugar which then triggers the stress response system and release of Cortisol. As we discussed, cortisol is released when needed to respond to stressful situations (running from a tiger), but in this case, the stress or emergency is low blood sugar. The last thing you need is to wake up in the middle of the night to go to the bathroom then lying awake for the next few hours feeling hungry and miserable. As you lie in bed worrying about not sleeping, your Cortisol increases making the problem worse. Best to avoid this in the first place by avoiding after dinner carbs and sugars (sorry folks this includes wine).

WHAT IS THE SOLUTION TO SLEEP BETTER AFTER EATING A MEAL?

First, know your metabolic type. Second, eat a balanced meal in the evening depending on your metabolic type. I recommend a spoonful of coconut oil before bedtime to help balance out your blood sugar. You can add this to herbal tea if the thought of a spoonful of oil gags you. Also, remember to eat right for your type throughout the day because your blood sugar levels could remain high for hours after eating too much sugar or carbs. I have spiked my blood sugar by eating too much fruit; even if I pour coconut oil over fresh berries and add heavy cream. Until you have a routine, I strongly urge you to test that blood sugar two hours after eating and stop eating two hours before bedtime.

THE NEW SLEEP MINDSET

After my experience with adrenal exhaustion and the impact on my sleep, I had a serious shift in my mindset on the importance of quality sleep and especially sleeping through the night. When you have adrenal burnout (adrenal fatigue or exhaustion, as I had experienced), the adrenals are exhausted and the cortisol and melatonin circadian rhythm is disrupted. Your hormone cortisol should be low during the night and increase around sunrise or 6:00 a.m. When you are dealing with high cortisol levels (known as Stage One and Stage Two adrenal fatigue), you find yourself wide awake around 2:00 a.m. staring at the ceiling.

Nowadays, I make sure I get my recommended seven to nine hours of sleep each night. I need eight to nine hours of sleep to wake up feeling refreshed and energized for my busy day ahead.

If you are "burning the candles at both ends" on a regular basis, you likely need an attitude adjustment and to make sleep a priority. While a strong work ethic is admirable, our society has trained us that to sit still is being lazy and to have an overbooked calendar is a sign of success. We sign up for extra activities just to add another gold star next to our name. We invent things to do (remodel after remodel for some) just to feel important. Some treat Shavasana at the end of power yoga as such a waste of precious time. This mindset requires a reset. Your health is your most important asset. Without it, your strong work ethic will do you no good. At some point, you will simply be unable to add activities that give you a gold star. Take some quiet time to reflect or journal about why you feel the need to be so busy. Is it to stave off anxiety? Feel important? Look successful to others? Remember that you are already important and that you matter in ways far beyond your busy life. If this section describes you then add "attitude adjustment" to your calendar. Just a few minutes each day can make it possible for you understand why you feel the need to stay so busy and to give yourself permission to slow down enough to get the sleep you need for a productive and healthy life.

If you try to get enough sleep and end up lying awake or waking throughout the night, it's time to do some sleep hacking and make the quality of sleep a priority. There are some basic "sleep hygiene" steps that can help improve your sleep quality.

A subset of these hacks include:

- Go to bed and wake up at the same time each night
- Sleep in as dark a room as you can (cover or remove LED clocks)
- Start winding down at least two hours before bed. This includes lowering the light and avoiding computers and TV.
- No coffee after 1:00 p.m.
- Go to bed no later than 11:00 p.m. (only if you can sleep until 7:00 a.m.)
- Goal is to go to bed by 10:00 p.m.
- No vigorous exercise within two hours of bedtime
- Put cell phones in airplane mode and preferably out of the room on the charger
- No Wi-Fi or wireless phones in the bedroom

These steps are reasonably simple to implement though it does not mean easy. Be gentle with yourself as you start to create new habits. If and when you do wake up at night, relax and watch your thoughts. Whatever you are worried about cannot be dealt with in the middle of the night. Visualize putting these issues in a drawer in your living room that you can open and look at when you get up in the morning. Count your breaths and know that just lying still gives your body some restful recovery. Know that due to sleep cycles (that we will cover next) you may lay awake for an hour or so until the next sleep cycle is due to kick in. When this happens try to lay still and watch your thoughts. Don't stress about not being able to sleep and know that at the next cycle you will fall asleep.

SLEEP STAGES

When we sleep, we typically move through five stages of sleep which make up our natural sleep cycle. Stages 1-4 are light to deep Non-Rapid Eye Movement (NREM) sleep while the 5th stage is known as and Rapid Eye Movement (REM) sleep. The average sleep cycle lasts 90 to 110 and the time spent in each stage varies as the night progresses. Overall, adults typically spend twenty to twenty-five percent (20-25%) of our time in REM sleep and the remaining time either awake or in NREM. Deeper sleep occurs mostly the first half of the night longer periods of (REM) the second half of the night. Waking may occur after REM sleep though if we are a good sleeper we may not even remember we were awake.

Each sleep stage has a host of characteristics including physical movements and muscle activity as well as the frequency and patterns of the brain waves. Sleep stages are monitored in a lab with an Electroencephalogram (a machine that measures brain waves) and a technician who visually monitors muscle and body movements. A summary of the sleep stages follows.

1. **Stage One:** This is where we are sleeping lightly, muscle activity slows down and occasional muscle twitching. This is four to five percent (4-5%) of our sleep. This is where we drift in and out of sleep and can be easily awakened while our eyes move slowly and muscle activity slows down. In this stage, you may have experienced sudden muscle contractions as if you are falling. I do this occasionally.

2. **Stage Two:** Our breathing pattern and heart rate slow down; we experience a slight decrease in body temperature. This is forty-five to fifty-five percent (45-55%) of our sleep. Our eye movement stops while our brain wave activity becomes slower with an occasional blast of rapid brain wave activity.

3. **Stage Three:** Deep sleep begins here and we start to generate slow delta waves. This is four to six percent (4-6%) of our sleep. The delta brain waves are interspersed with smaller faster brain waves. Delta waves are associated with the deepest levels of relaxation and restoration... a more healing stage of sleep. Delta brainwaves help us feel rejuvenated when we wake up in after a solid night's sleep.

4. **Stage Four:** This is where we transition into a very deep sleep with more rhythmic breathing with no eye movement and limited muscle activity. We start to produce more delta brain waves almost exclusively. This is twelve to fifteen percent (12-15%) of our sleep. Sleep stages three and four are referred to as deep sleep or more of delta brainwave sleep. This is when it is more difficult to be awakened.

5. **Stage Five:** REM Period or rapid eye movement; brain waves speed up and we start dreaming. Muscles relax and the heart rate increases while our breathing is rapid. Irregular and shallow. Our eyes move rapidly and our muscles are more still while the heart rate and blood pressure increase. This is twenty to twenty-five percent (20-25%)

of our sleep. The REM stage is when we dream the most during sleep – and we may remember the dreams if we awaken during this period. It has been reported that most people experience around three to five intervals of this REM sleep stage each night.

We sleep for recovery, physical repair, psychological repair, growth, renewal, and restoration. Each stage of sleep offers various benefits for our body and mind including a surge of growth hormones during our first cycle of deep sleep. We need each stage: light sleep, deep sleep, and REM sleep stages. As we age, we get less deep sleep and more time in light sleep... as we say to sleep like a baby is to have plenty of deep sleep. When we wake up feeling refreshed, we may have gotten more deep sleep as previous nights.

Other processes that occur while we sleep are important for the body to recovery and repair. Proper recovery helps improve performance for life and sports. Recovery time, while we sleep, offers a restful state for the body while cell growth and rebuilding occur.

While the need for sleep is still somewhat a mystery, some hypotheses developed by scientists on why humans require sleep each night (and can go without food more than they can survive without sleep) include:

- By removing the stimulus one receives while awake, the brain can reorder. It has a chance to exercise important neuronal connections that might otherwise deteriorate due to lack of activity.
- Sleep gives the brain an opportunity to reorganize data to help find a solution to the problem, process newly learned information, and organize and archive memories.
- Sleep is a time for serious rest. Sleep lowers a person's metabolic rate and energy consumption. The allostatic load (or "daily wear and tear") on the body takes a toll and sleep is a respite.
- The cardiovascular system also gets a break during sleep. Researchers have found that people with normal or high blood pressure experience a twenty to thirty percent (20-30%) reduction in blood pressure and ten to twenty percent (10-20%) reduction in heart rate.
- During sleep, the body has a chance to replace chemicals and repair muscles, other tissues, and aging or dead cells. Growth hormones are released during deep sleep.
-

BRAIN WAVES

Brain waves are the result of interaction between our neurons within our brains and are produced by the synchronized electrical pulses from masses of neurons communicating with each other. Like most electrical signals, these brainwaves have an amplitude and frequency and are divided into *bandwidths* to describe their functions.

Our brainwaves change according to what we're doing and feeling. When slower brainwaves are dominant, we can feel tired, slow, sluggish, or dreamy. The higher frequencies are dominant when we feel wired, or alert. To summarize the brain frequency wave range:

BETA: The beta waves are low amplitude brainwaves between 12 – 38 Hz and are most common when we are awake, conscious thought, logical thinking, and stimulating effect. Beta waves allow us to focus and complete tasks easily. Too much beta wave can lead to excessive stress and anxiety. For some, this can be due to consuming too much coffee or caffeine.

ALPHA: The alpha brain waves (8 - 12Hz) have a higher amplitude than Beta and are associated with calm thoughts or a meditative state. The brain is quite receptive and open to suggestion in the Alpha state. Be aware that watching TV puts most people into the Alpha state and that advertisers and other propaganda machines take full advantage of this. When we become stressed or anxious, we may experience what some call alpha blocking (which when the beta brain waves block out alpha brain wave activity) as we become overstimulated or too stressed. Ideally, we are feeling a deep sense of relaxation when we are in alpha, a stage we need to be in more frequently during the day.

THETA: The optimal amount of Theta brain waves (3 - 8Hz) will bring us into the creative mind, emotional connection, intuitiveness, and relaxation. This frequency range is connected to daydreaming and sleeping. In Theta waves, we experience and feel deep emotions. An interesting piece of information is that too much Theta wave can bring people to be depressed, deeply relaxed semi-hypnotic state, as well as increased ADHD, hyperactivity, and impulsiveness. On the other end of the spectrum, too little time in theta waves can be connected to anxiety, stress, and

79

poor emotional awareness.

DELTA: The delta waves (.5 – 3Hz) are where we improve our immune system and natural healing while in restorative deep sleep. We all need this brainwave during our sleep cycle, but many people miss time at this stage due to sleep challenges (stress and sugar). We experienced more time in Delta when we were infants and as a younger child, though we tend to spend less time here as we age. This brainwave frequency is when we are in the deepest stage of our sleep. Delta waves are involved with unconscious body functions as heart rate regulation and digestion. When we have spent enough time in Delta, we wake up feeling refreshed and rejuvenated.

One of my podcast interviews with Dr. Phil Maffetone involved a discussion on the stages of sleep and brain waves (episode 70 on my Fit Fat Fast Podcast). We talked about how you should be able to get into Alpha Brain Wave State while exercising. This is often referred to as "in the zone" during a run or bike ride and is a form of a meditative state. This is where we lose track of time and become immersed in the flow of the activity.

Dr. Maffetone shares his explanations of the five brain waves, the state of consciousness and how to get into alpha brainwave state. When we are trying to fall asleep we need to shut the mind off and feel calm and relaxed. Unfortunately, I hear most clients struggle (including myself in the past) with a busy mind and feeling wired. A solution to this is to lie down, be still, and focus on deep breathing as long slow deep breathing techniques can help us get into Alpha brain waves. Also, listening to calm meditative music can help you can get into this Alpha wave state in less than five minutes. You can also use these techniques if you need to take a pause and reset break during the afternoon or anytime you feel exhausted and tired but wired.

I go to sleep now with my Sonos music timer set for one to two hours. I play yoga, relaxation, or calm meditative type of music to help prepare my mind for bedtime. I found this prep for sleep really has improved my quality of sleep and allows for me to get into Alpha state before I doze off. Dr. Phil Maffetone has a great lesson on his website called Five Minute Power Break you can implement into your lifestyle any time of the day (http://tinyurl.com/5MinutePowerBreak).

If you take forty to sixty minutes to fall asleep or if you fall asleep then you wake up around 2:00 a.m., it is a problem. If you can't fall asleep, you may be stuck in beta waves and thinking about your to-do list or your day or obsessing about something that, at that moment, you can do absolutely nothing about. The goal is to learn to let go and get some rest and address your issues the next do when you actually *can* do something about them. There are various reasons besides mental chatter that are keeping you awake. It could be too little Vitamin D or calcium deficiency. If you are stuck in Beta and can't make Alpha waves, it could even be related to an accident that resulted in whiplash, per Dr. Maffetone, which has impaired Alpha production.

Dr. Maffetone suggests starting from the top down to relax starting with a healthy body and a healthy brain. Making the brain healthy will assist with your sleep functions. By eating healthy fats (the brain is sixty percent (60%) fat), moderate proteins, and avoiding sugar (not to spike insulin levels) we can assist the brain to function optimally. If we don't eat good fats, the brain doesn't work as well. Also, if we eat too much sugar, it is not good for the brain. A healthy brain is more able to function properly in many ways, including producing the desired brain waves for sleep.

SLEEP AND HEART RATE VARIABILITY

As we see, physical, chemical, nutritional, mental, and emotional states can result in out of sync brain waves and keep you wired when you should be tired. As we discussed in previous chapter Heart Rate Variability (HRV) is an excellent way to monitor your nervous system and is a great tool to hack your way to better health and better sleep. Since your brain is connected to the Autonomic Nervous System, HRV is an indication of whether the neurons in your brain are in an optimal state. If you have done too much physical training or overstimulate the sympathetic nervous system without allowing the parasympathetic nervous system kick in to help balance the overload on the nervous system, you can end up in chronic "Fight or Flight" and an overactive HPA axis. Over time, if you don't allow enough recovery time, the brain is exposed to too much sympatric and not enough parasympathetic stimulus.

While the adrenals are trying to keep up with your non-stop stress or extra activity, the brain is aware that you are beating yourself up with stress. The more you ignore the red flags of doing too much without resting, the more your body compensates by releasing more cortisol, reduced testosterone, estrogens, and other hormones to help keep up with the production of stress hormones. What does this have to do with sleep? Too much stress is involved in each of the eight elements of The WHOLESTIC Method.

Ronda Collier came on *The WHOLE Athlete* podcast to chat about the relationship between heart rate variability, sleep, and recovery for athletes of all levels. We talked about how sleep is important for one's health and discussed the HPA axis.

Human sleep is directly related to the level of stress which can result in adrenal fatigue issue.

Our sympathetic nervous system activates the flight and fight hormones including cortisol. If we are being chased by a tiger, the fight and flight emergency response system in the body—the stress hormones—are activated until the tiger is gone or killed. Once the threat subsides, we literally shake off the accumulated energy. If you have ever been in an accident, you may know firsthand about the body shaking after the event. In modern living traffic jams, our bosses, having children, etc. are all stressors. The end result is we are in a permanent state of fight and flight and do not "shake off" the accumulated stress energy. In addition, we rarely take the time to recover from our daily stress, usually due to our constant busy schedules and fast moving life which leaves us living in a state of the chronic fight and flight patterns.

When we activate our sympathetic nervous system which then causes activation of HPA Axis (hypothalamus-pituitary-adrenal axis), our stress hormones are released to respond to the situation including the hormone cortisol. When hypothalamus gets triggered, it causes CRH hormone to be released which acts directly on pituitary releasing ACTH (adrenocorticotropic hormone) also known as one of the stress hormones. ACTH travels through the bloodstream and acts on adrenal gland resulting in cortisol release, which is an inhibitor of ACTH and CRH. This whole mechanism of the cascade is what is called feedback loop mechanism.

Heart Rate Variability (HRV) is the perfect way to measure and manage stress (and overtraining). As Lord Kelvin said, "If you can't measure it, you can't improve it."

HRV measures a few metrics:
- The power and balance of the Autonomic Nervous System branches
- Vagal Tone

Not only does the balance of the Sympathetic and Parasympathetic nervous system matter, the "Power" of the nervous systems matters, as well. Consider a stereo receiver. A 50-watt receiver will reach distortion at high volumes whereas a 250-watt receiver will play clean music at much higher volumes. It turns out that HRV can measure the power of your nervous system giving you the tools to learn about what activities power you up or wear you down. The balance refers to a nervous system that is not dominated by one branch or another. Like left and right speakers, we want balance when we listen. Occasionally, the stereo aspect kicks in and we hear an instrument in one speaker or the other while overall the speakers both seem to be playing equally. When you have a balanced and powerful nervous system you are able to take on more without distortion (also known as stress and breakdown).

The *Vagus Nerve* is the tenth of twelve cranial nerves which and is involved in mediating the heart rate to slow it down. Strong vagal tone helps to counter the effects of fight or flight by decreasing heart rate and allowing the Parasympathetic branch to do its thing. When Vagal Tone is low, Cortisol may be allowed to run amok which, as we have described, impacts sleep.

A few ways to use HRV to hack sleep include taking your HRV before bed and upon waking or recording your HRV all night while you sleep. Ronda recommends the all-night HRV hack so you can get a bird's eye view of what is going on while you sleep. Your HRV should slowly and steadily increase throughout the night. If it does not, something is amiss. While sleep stage estimation using popular wearables is amusing; what really matters is whether the body repaired and recovered during sleep, and HRV will provide that feedback. As we will see in the next section that it is best to put your phone in airplane mode while you are asleep, you can still turn on the Bluetooth and then use SweetBeatHRV to monitor you HRV when your phone is in airplane mode.

A reason for taking it before bed and upon waking is illustrated by one of Ronda's clients who was waking up exhausted even though she thought she was getting good night's sleep. To hack this, she measured her nighttime and following morning HRV. What she found was that her HRV actually went down after sleeping 8 hours. She worked with Ronda and SweetWater Health and it was suggested that she was allergic or sensitive to something in her bed. The next few nights she slept in the spare room and her HRV increase as it should after 8 hours of sleep. Together they were able to determine that she was sensitive to something in her bed and her client went on to isolate the culprit by removing bedding one at a time while checking night and morning HRV. It turned out to be her comforter and noticed it was going down.

WIRELESS AND SLEEP

Ronda shared that she is a good sleeper because she has put stress out of her life. She has been doing meditation since 2005 and yoga for more than twenty years. While for the most part, her sleep is good, she noticed she kept waking up suddenly during the night and then going right back to sleep. After doing some deep internet digging, she learned about how exposure to microwave frequencies such as Wi-Fi and Cell Phones, can impact our health in many ways, including sleep disruption.

Would you get inside a microwave oven and press start? Of course not. However, most people are receiving a heavy dose of electromagnetic fields all day and all night - some are of their choosing and others are not. Microwave frequencies include a range from 300 MHz to 300 GHz. Wi-Fi frequency is 2.4 GHz, 4G Cell Phone frequency is 1.9 GHz and for those who still have a landline and cordless phones you are looking at 1.9 GHz. In addition, you may not even realize that your utility smart meter that was installed without your permission transmits between 902 MHz and 2.4 GHz and transmits pulses at a rate of 2–20/second. Many people who live in apartments that share a wall with the multiple utility units became quite sick and with severe sleep disruption once the smart meters were installed. Oh did I mention the utility companies can tell when you are home by your usage and that they sell that data to advertisers?

I digress.

While the power output of these devices is claimed to be safe there is a study concluding by the National Toxicology Program that will provide more information, though the preliminary report shows an increase in cancer in rats with heavy exposure. Relatively little is known about the safety of microwave exposure and we are the guinea pigs. It is hypothesized that these frequencies interrupt cellular communication which is No Bueno for living organisms and can create a host of health issues, including sleep disruption.

When Ronda learned this she changed to wired Ethernet for internet and turned off her home Wi-Fi. She opted out of the smart meter and since she still had a landline with wireless handsets she replaced them with wired phones. In addition, she removed any electronics from her bedside table and if they were in the room, she turns them off or put them in airplane mode. After doing all that, the sudden hourly waking pattern transformed to a normal pattern and a good night's sleep.

SUMMARY OF SLEEP HACKS

In summary, there are many things you can do to improve your sleep. For many, this will take discipline to implement the good sleep hygiene techniques. These are new habits and old habits, as we know, can be hard to break. You may some smartphone applications that will help and which can be set to wake you up near your desired time while allowing you to complete your current sleep cycle.

Here are some sleep hacks so you can sleep like a baby:

1. Wind down before bedtime. Start by avoiding electronic devices one to three hours before bed, including computer, iPad, and cell phones. Instead, you can focus on relaxing, unwinding, and reading.
2. If you must use these devices, purchase some inexpensive blue filter glasses to filter the sleep delaying blue light.

3. Minimize exposure to bright lights two hours before bed by trying to use dimmer switch controls, low wattage lights, or even candles.

4. Sleep ideally from 10:00 p.m. to 6:00 a.m. and wake up naturally with the sunrise. Remember, your repair and restore cycles occur while you are asleep. Sleep more if you have any injuries, immune issue, depression, headaches, or fatigue.

5. Create a dark room and environment to sleep in each night. Black out your room and eliminate any flashing lights. I cover my alarm clock lights, air conditioner, and anything else that emits light. Keep your room cool and have a fan on to help your quality of sleep.

6. During The WHOLESTIC Method coaching program, try wearing a sleep tracking device such as a Fitbit or use a sleep app (put the phone on airplane mode) to track the quality of sleep and movement during the night. Do an overnight HRV session.

7. Avoid eating too much sugar in the evening, including fruit. Sugars will disrupt sleep cycles by spiking up blood sugar levels. Review the nutrition section to learn how to eat right for your metabolic type. Try eating 1-2 tablespoons of coconut oil or MCT C8 oil before bed if you are actually hungry at bedtime and do not want to spike blood sugar levels which will disrupt circadian rhythm.

8. Be cautious of what type of exercise you do close to bedtime. Too much high-intensity interval training or chronic cardio sessions may disrupt your sleep cycle and can increase your cortisol levels. Instead, try lower intensity exercise such as a walk, Pilates, or yoga in the evenings.

9. Avoid stimulants such as coffee and other caffeinated beverages after lunchtime or 1:00 p.m. Caffeine has a half-life of six hours, so if you have coffee too late in the day, you will disrupt your physical, immune, and psychological repair cycles. You definitely do not want to stimulate your adrenal glands in the evening or during sleep cycle which results in cortisol released when it should be suppressed.

10. Hydrate throughout the day - not at all at night. Remember to drink half your body weight in ounces to stay hydrated and add some sea salt if you are not retaining your water.

11. Try some natural herbal supplements to help you sleep. Chamomile or Valerian root tea; GABA, L-Dopa, Magnesium, or other suggestions from your naturopath or functional medicine doctor.

12. If you can't turn off your mind, try deep breathing exercises by counting inhales and matching the length of your exhales. Focus on each breath.

13. If you can, give yourself at least one morning a week to wake up on your own, without an alarm.

14. Power naps in the afternoons for fifteen to thirty-minutes work wonders.

15. Get off your sleep meds. Too much dependency on a drug that probably isn't helping, as well as having adverse side effects, is not worth the trouble.

16. Try some essential oils in a diffuser or on your neck such as lavender, chamomile, or peppermint oils.

17. Get a massage chair or recovery boots at the Norma-Tech or even try a bath with Epsom salts and essential oils such as lavender.

18. Write in your gratitude journal before bed to reduce stress and worries from the day. Write your goals for the next day for your to-do list.

19. Track your heart rate variability in the morning to monitor your quality of sleep as you should wake up feeling rested and re-energized.

20. Starting tonight, I want you to get seven to nine hours of solid sleep per night. When you let these natural boosts occur during sleep, you'll wake up refreshed and reenergized for the day ahead.

Reviewing the circadian clock, you can see the ideal time for sexual activity, coordination/reaction time sports, cardiovascular, and strength workouts, as well as ideal time to be in bed:

6:00 a.m. - wake up around sunrise
6:45 a.m. - the sharpest rise in blood pressure
7:30 a.m. - Melatonin secretion stops
8:30 a.m. - Bowel movement likely
9:00 a.m. - highest testosterone secretion
10:00 a.m. - High Alertness
12:00 p.m.
2:30 p.m. - Best coordination
3:30 p.m. - Fastest reaction time
5:00 p.m. - Greatest cardiovascular efficiency and muscle strength
6:30 p.m. - Highest blood pressure
7:00 p.m. - Highest body temperature
9:00 p.m. - Melatonin secretion starts
10:30 p.m. -Bowel movement suppressed
12:00 a.m.

2:00 a.m. - Deepest Sleep
4:30 a.m. - Lowest body temperature

My friend, Brock, and I did a fun podcast about the importance of sleep on *The WHOLE Athlete*. We discussed the importance of sleep for fitness and weight control. We both agree there isn't nearly enough attention paid to sleeping as an important component of a healthy lifestyle.

Sleep is an important part of training, fitness, weight management, and life in general. Unfortunately, it tends to be the first thing we sacrifice to achieve other goals. As part of our go-go lifestyle, we'll always cut into our sleep time to get more time to do whatever is our top priority.

A significant aspect of sleep often forgotten is the importance of sleep for weight management (*read my past blog post about sleep and weight loss below*). Sleep affects the hormone levels in your body, mainly those controlling when you feel hungry or full. See the WebMD article about hunger hormones and sleep for another article on the way that sleep affects metabolism.

In the end, Brock pointed out one of the most important things about improving your sleeping is when you find yourself lying awake don't get stressed about sleeping. Being stressed is certain to keep you awake. So, while sleeping is definitely something worth thinking about, avoid letting it give you stress since that will almost certainly lead to even less sleep.

We need to find the right balance of the nervous system between stress hormones and repair hormones. Too much of one or the other causes imbalance in our hormonal system and we know where that goes.

What is the right amount for you to be in equilibrium?

The big five WHOLESTIC Method Sleep tips for becoming a fat burner:

1. _____
2. _____
3. _____
4. _____
5. _____

The WHOLESTIC Method to improving fat loss, health and performance for life and sports by working from the inside out.

REFERENCES:

www.adrenalfatiguerecovery.com/sleep-and-stress

http://tinyurl.com/SleepPerfAndRecvry

www.chekinstitute.com

www.superhumancoach.com

https://web.mst.edu/psyworld/sleep_stages.htm

http://www.sleepdex.org/stages.htm

http://tinyurl.com/ChronicTiredness

http://tinyurl.com/BloodSugarAndSleep

http://tinyurl.com/TooMuchTooLittle

http://tinyurl.com/BrainWaveTypes

http://tinyurl.com/DrLamTiredness

http://tinyurl.com/BrainwaveOverview

http://tinyurl.com/SleepModMetabolism

http://tinyurl.com/SleedAndWeightLoss

ELEMENT #4
STRESS

Everyone feels stressed from time to time... but what is stress, and how does it impact our ability to be fat burners and maintain overall health and wellbeing?

In this chapter, we will look at the fundamental stress response and its purpose, the connection between mental and physical stress, the different types of stress (SAM vs. HPA vs. Eustress), and what we can do about it.

Stress is the root of most people's health problems, but they are unaware of it. Every day, people juggle a busy schedule, family, and life obligations. Then, we add a full training schedule for a 50K, marathon, or Ironman distance triathlon or we have a tragic death in our family, lose a job, or get divorce papers.

What does the stress do to your body... your gut, your joints, and your brain? We will explore these issues in this chapter.

SAM, HPA, AND EUSTRESS

Throughout human evolution, the stress response has been critical to survival. When our hunter-gatherer ancestors came across a saber-tooth tiger (or other clear and present danger) the Sympathetic-Adrenal-Medullary (SAM) stress response, also known as the "Fight or Flight" response kicked in. Within seconds it primed the body to either run away from the threat or fight it out.

Physiologically, when a threat is perceived amygdala sends a distress signal and the hypothalamus activates the sympathetic nervous system with then stimulates the adrenal medulla resulting in the release of adrenaline and noradrenaline. This sympathetic nervous system overdrive causes an increase in the heart rate, blood pressure, and breathing rate. The skin temperature decreases as blood flow is diverted to the muscles (and the part of the brain that controls the muscles), digestion is shut down (who needs to digest when you may not live another 5 minutes), and the pupils dilate to increase visual input. This explains why, after a fright, we may be pale with pounding heart, wide eyes and feeling jittery.

Once the threat is over, our ancestors would literally shake it off. This is a natural mechanism to discharge the muscular tension and reset our systems back to baseline. Many of us have felt this trembling after an accident though most do not realize that this is literally shaking off the stress response. If this tension is not shaken out, then signals are sent to the brain that we are still under threat which causes us to tighten up even more and a vicious cycle ensues.

While the SAM stress response is associated with short-term or acute stress, the Hypothalamic-Pituitary-Adrenal (HPA) is activated by chronic stress. Long-term stressors such as worry about work, children, or relationships can invoke the HPA stress response (which usually takes twenty minutes to kick in). Physiologically the hypothalamus releases CRF with stimulates the pituitary gland to release ACTH, stimulating the adrenal cortex with then produces corticosteroids. These stimulate the liver to release energy for dealing with the ongoing threat.

We love to be busy, overscheduled, and race through the day, but our addiction to being busy could be causing us to be chronically stressed with an overactive HPA stress response. This can make us fat and struggle to lose weight. Remember, chronic stress can cause cortisol dysregulation. Too much of anything is toxic and leads to dysregulation in the body, including sleep and your thyroid. The excessive activation of cortisol can affect the thyroid function because cortisol inactivates T3 thyroid hormone and shunts it into reverse T3 which then results in thyroid problems.

If thyroid hormones are low and the body perceives stress, the HPA Axis is activated and the stress hormone cortisol is released. We can get ourselves into a non-stop cycle which can make one insane. Once chronic thyroid and cortisol dysregulation happens, this can activate adrenaline acting as a substitute for cortisol which can result in a more dreadful panic feeling. So, this is a reason many people wake up at 3:00-4:00 a.m. in a panic state and can't go back to sleep again. Dysfunctional HPA Axis activity may play a role in some sleep disorders, but in other cases, HPA dysfunction is the result of poor sleep or sleep disorders, so it's all an interconnected thing.

Here is a chart to demonstrate the stress response system of the HPA Axis. Permission to use from www.adrenalfatiguesolution.com

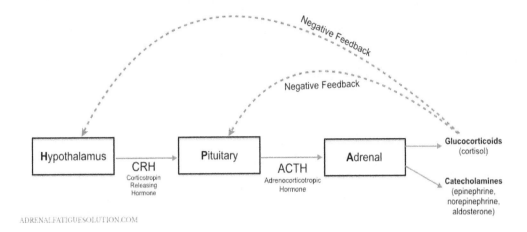

ADRENALFATIGUESOLUTION.COM

Chronic stress will not only mess with your hormones, it also disrupts your natural cortisol levels that shift throughout the day and regulate your circadian rhythm.

A broken circadian rhythm will cause your metabolism to slow and will:

- Raise your blood sugar
- Reduce your ability to burn fat
- Increase your hunger levels and sugar cravings
- Cause hormonal imbalances
- Increase belly fat and create fatty liver
- Increase the rate at which you store fat
- Raise the level of fatty acids and triglycerides in your blood

Eustress is a term that psychologists have coined to describe positive and motivating stress. This type of stress can be experienced as enthusiasm and drive and is usually self-imposed. However, if periods of eustress continue without pause, it can turn into chronic HPA type stress response, and this spells trouble.

THE AUTONOMIC NERVOUS SYSTEM AND STRESS

As we have discussed in previous chapters, the Autonomic Nervous System (ANS) consists of two main branches, the Sympathetic and Parasympathetic. The sympathetic nervous system prepares the body for intense physical activity and controls the body's response to a perceived. On the flip side, the parasympathetic nervous system does the opposite by controlling homeostasis, relaxing the body, and slowing down high energy functions.

The importance of the parasympathetic nervous system (PNS) is often ignored. Instead, we give more of our attention to the sympathetic nervous system and the flight or fight go-go-go lifestyle. Most of us are a little short in the rest and digest department, at least from my observations of clients and friends. Most people do not know that the PNS can be strengthened. So let's talk about *Vagal Tone*.

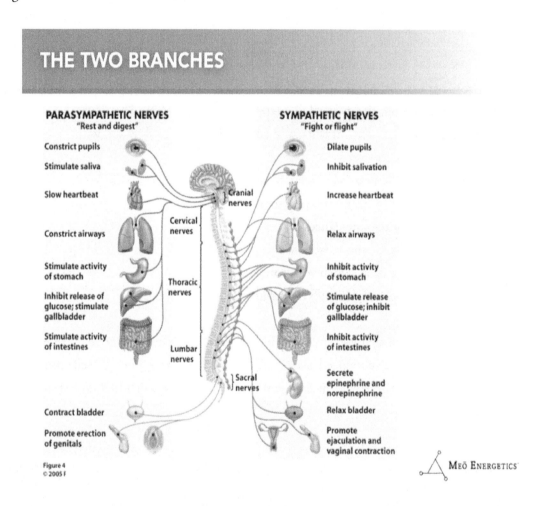

Figure 4
© 2005 F

MEŌ ENERGETICS

The Vagus Nerve is the tenth of twelve cranial nerves and is a major mediator of the PNS. The strength of the vagus nerve is called vagal tone and we can do exercises (discussed next) to strengthen this vagal tone. How does this help? When the SNS kicks in and we enter a stressful situation, a strong vagal tone provides the capability of "calming down" the SAM fight or flight response. In addition, vagus nerve stimulation normalizes an elevate HPA axis.

In the chapter on stress in Paul Chek's Eat, Move and Be Healthy book, he explains the different kinds of stress. I interviewed C.H.E.K Practitioner, Jator Pierre, to explain the types of stress we have in our lives including internal and external stressors:

The sympathetic nervous system and the parasympathetic nervous system are activated with repeated stress that hits us every day. We all deal and react to stress differently. We have two parts of our automatic nervous system; sympathetic nervous systems (SNS) produce the flight-or-fight nervous response. A stressful situation will activate the SNS as your fight or flight... then your body responds by releasing stress hormones to increase your sweat rate, heart rate, and blood pressure. The redirection of the blood is shunted away from your internal organs to the skin and muscles then reduces the digestive and elimination processes of the body in response to the stress. When the SNS is over-activated, the hormone cortisol levels are increased which results in the suppression of the growth and repair hormones. The body begins to break down muscle tissue and increases fatigue as the cortisol levels are increased over a long period of time (faucet keeps running) which leads to dysfunction of the immune system.

When the parasympathetic nervous system (PNS) is suppressed... we have digestion and repair problems as well as hormone dysfunction since the PNS stimulates digestion, metabolism as well as the release of tissue building hormones.

We need to find the right balance of the nervous system... the balance between stress hormones and repair hormones. Too much of one or the other causes an imbalance in our hormonal system.

I also spoke with Sweetwater Health CEO, Ronda Collier, about how to measure and monitor your stress levels using the SweetBeatHRV app. She noted that the status of the Nervous System is an important indicator of acute or chronic stress. As we have already learned, Heart Rate Variability (HRV) is a view of the autonomic nervous system and thus can be used to monitor daily stress levels. She made an important point that the brain is a giant pattern matcher and the brain filters out what is familiar over time. Otherwise, you would be constantly aware of your shirt on your skin. While this filtering has huge benefits, the downside is it will filter anything familiar even if it is dysfunctional. Therefore, many people have chronic stress and don't know it because they have acclimated to feeling that way. This is why measuring your nervous system is so important.

Personalized health and medicine are increasingly important as stress levels increase with our busy lifestyles. Stress is the weak link in the chain and is responsible for more than ninety percent (90%) of diseases. The SweetBeatHRV app measures:

- SNS Power – LF value in app
- PNS Power – HF value in app
- Vagal Tone – HRV Value in app
- SNS-PNS Ratio – LF/HF value in app
- Stress level from relaxed blue to stressed red

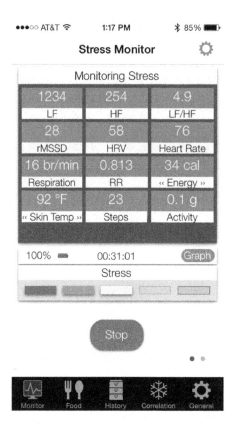

Many different influences can induce stress, from internal worries to stress on the body caused by exertion or surgery. This can cause your HRV to be low, your SNS/PNS (LF/HF) to be very high (>6) indicating a dominant fight or flight response. Also, HRV can vary due to several different factors, including age, gender, disease, or stress, among many other things.

The SweetBeatHRV app allows you to be your own health advocate and guide yourself as it measures your stress response by measuring the autonomic nervous system sympathetic and parasympathetic branches (and the balance between them) as well as vagal tone.

SweetBeatHRV gives you so much more information than only your heart rate variability (HRV) including your correlations to other apps to give you meaningful information from all the data you have been collecting or tracking. When you are training for an event or race, you can use the feedback from your SweetBeatHRV measurements to help you train smart, perform better, and lose fat weight. Get some insight on your health, especially if you are training for a race or leading an overscheduled stressed life. Not one size fits all. Visit www.SweetWaterHRV.com for more information.

STRESS MANAGEMENT TECHNIQUES

I remember when I was first married to my husband, Neal, and we visited his parents in Tucson. They were aware of my participation in Ironman Triathlons—not sure if they knew what they involved, but they knew I did a lot of exercises. My father-in-law took me into the family room and opened a page in a book by Andrew Weil, I forget exactly what the paragraph said, but it had something to do with how excessive exercise can impact your ability to get pregnant. (I guess he really wanted grandchildren.) At the time, I thought the exercise I was doing was not impacting my health, but as you will find out, endurance exercise, also known as chronic cardio, is another form of stress. Too much of any type of stress may impact our health and lead to hormonal imbalances. My father-in-law was on to my busy non-stop personality. I never could get pregnant.

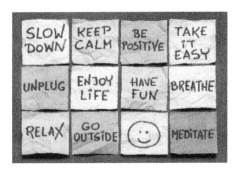

In *Life is Not a Race,* you'll learn from my personal experience of trying to accomplish too much in one day every day for years and then add in training for Ironman distance Triathlons, marathons, and 50K trail runs. We can't be invincible and try to be over-achievers every day or else you reach a breaking point that creates a domino effect in your internal health communication system and command center—the HPA axis. More is not better and that includes our daily lifestyle and training habits. Less is more. We need to learn how to disconnect to connect with ourselves to decompress, re-energize, and recalibrate.

We need to learn how to take a stroll, hum, or sing while driving and whistle while we walk, as my grandpa used to do as I was growing up. I discovered I was always tense... or intense. What is the opposite of being too tense or intense? Maybe relaxed, at ease, and laid back? What is the right balance of passion, dedication, and intensity without leading to anxiety? Are we able to be at ease, low-key, and calm without being lazy? I say yes.

As I have discovered from my own experience of living each day as a race and in my new journey transforming into a WHOLE Athlete, we don't need to train long hours, multiple days, and at high heart rates that often lead to burnout and breakdown.

Mark Allen talked about his career as a triathlete and his connection with Brant Secunda, a shaman, healer, and ceremonial leader of the Huichol people. Together, they are co-authors of the book, *Fit Soul, Fit Body: 9 Keys to a Healthier Happier You*. Mark runs www.fitsoul-fitbody.com and Brant's website is at www.shamanism.com.

Mark talks about the value of connecting to nature in your training. His attraction to the Ironman was at least partly inspired by his love for the big island of Hawaii. Since then, he's found some answers to his questions of how to make training a joy rather than a chore and what was

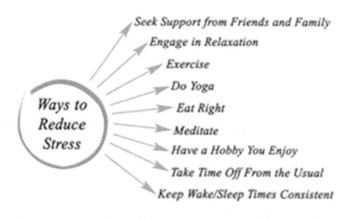

driving him to do endurance sports.

He talks in our *The WHOLE Athlete* podcast about the importance of training as a lifestyle; so, it's naturally a part of what you do every day. He emphasizes that training needs to improve health rather than simply be a burden. His philosophy emphasizes the mind and body connection in training rather than being simply a mechanical process to improve muscle mass or speed.

He also discusses the keys to improved happiness from his book because, yes, happiness is another element connected to stress:

Ways to Reduce Stress

- Seek Support from Friends and Family
- Engage in Relaxation
- Exercise
- Do Yoga
- Eat Right
- Meditate
- Have a Hobby You Enjoy
- Take Time Off From the Usual
- Keep Wake/Sleep Times Consistent

- Quiet your mind and manage your stress
- Make a connection to the spiritual world in nature
- Manage the different types of stress
- Know and set your quest. Understand why you do the things you do.
- Live what you ask for
- Slow down to get faster
- Invite your inner caveman to the table as far as diet goes.

Read more from Mark Allen on http://www.fitsoul-fitbody.com, as he is known for his success in Ironman when he learned how to quiet his mind and focus from the inside out.

You may not necessarily be able to eliminate the causes of stress, but there are ways to reduce its negative impact. One is to do what we call in our book, Quieting the Mind. There is an entire key devoted to this. In tough moments, often the only thing that can be changed are the thoughts that are running through our brains, and usually, they are not the ones that help us out. But, if we practice quieting the mind, then at least we can give ourselves a break from our own internal chatter, which often opens the space to hear the answers and solutions we are working so hard to find.

Then, in addition to this, use nature as a source of stress reduction and personal inspiration. Walk in the woods, sit by a stream, jump in the ocean, and breathe in the colors of the sunset. These are all tools Brant has us do in workshops he leads. Every single one can give you a calmer feel inside and reinvigorate your trust in life. It sounds simple, and it is, but it can also be a powerful tool for bringing a healthy and happy attitude back when you may not feel it so strongly.

HOW CAN YOU MANAGE YOUR STRESS?

Here are a few solutions I give my clients to implement into their lives:
- Select healthy food when you have the urge to eat sugar. Mix a teaspoon of raw almond butter with a teaspoon of coconut oil to curb your cravings or if you need something crunchy then try cut up celery and cucumbers.
- Avoid caffeine and sugar.
- Change your reaction to a stressful situation by going for a walk and process the information before you act or respond.

- Deep, slow, breathing exercises are simple to do while you are stuck in traffic or feeling anxious.
- Deep Breathing at a 2:1 Exhale-to-Inhale ratio is shown to balance the nervous system and strengthen the vagal tone.
- Avoid over-scheduling your day and leave extra time between appointments or meetings so you are not feeling rushed.
- Schedule time for yourself each day.
- Alternate hard workout days with easy days or eliminate hard workouts if overstressed as they will be counterproductive.
- Practice the tips from our previous chapter on improving your sleep.
- Measure your HRV
  - When you see stress levels from moment to moment, you can also change what you are doing or thinking to reduce stress. Conscious breathing exercises balance the nervous system, and therefore you will see an immediate rise in HRV.
  - Some may prefer to meditate, exercise, or do yoga—but whatever stress reduction method you employ, now you have real-time feedback, enabling you to take charge of reducing stress. Long-term behavioral modifications, including sustained fitness and good nutrition, will also reduce chronic stress. SweetBeat also allows you to upload your sessions to a secure database, where your data feeds into a personal calendar.
  - You can see throughout a given day, week, or month exactly when your stress levels are highest, allowing you to be proactive in addressing stress-creation. For example, if your recorded sessions show that commute time is always highly stressful, you might choose to play relaxing music during the drive instead of listening to the news on the radio. The Sweetwater Health website offers links to our health partners, who offer a variety of approaches to stress reduction ranging from fitness to meditation and yoga.

ESSENTIAL OILS

Recently I started experimenting with essential oils to help with relaxation and recovery through a new friend, Marylou, who specializes with essential oils in her holistic coaching program.

If you have ever enjoyed the scent of a flower, you've experienced the aromatic qualities of essential oils. These naturally occurring, volatile aromatic compounds are found in the bark, stems, flowers, roots, and other parts of a plant. Essential oils give a plant its distinctive smell, protect the plant, and play a role in its pollination. In addition to their intrinsic benefits to plants and their amazing fragrance, essential oils have long been used by humans as plant-based medicine.

The physical and chemical properties of the volatile aromatic compounds that compose essential oils allow them to quickly move through the air and directly interact with the olfactory sensors in the nose. Such unique properties make essential oils ideal for aromatherapy—using these compounds from plants to help maintain a healthy mind and body—as well as topical applications. The type of compounds present in an essential oil determines the oil's aroma and the benefits it has for the user. Essential oils can be used for a wide range of emotional and physical wellness applications and make great non-toxic versions of cleaning products and air fresheners.

The leaves of the tree were for the healing of the nations.
Rev. 22:2

Essential oils are our passion here at Awesome Natural Healing. These beautiful Biblical oils are truly God's medicine. He made us so perfectly and He gave us wonderful foods to nourish us and the oils from his powerful plant life to keep our body thriving, physically and emotionally. When you are ready to add essential oils to your wellness routine and replace toxic medicines, toxic cleaners, and toxic air fresheners with these amazing oils, we are here to help you.

Marylou and I met online in our Dr. Josh Axe Institute of Nutritional Leadership course. She is a holistic lifestyle coach and passionate about helping others heal their bodies from the inside out. Learn more at www.draxe.com/essential-oil-uses-benefits.

WHAT ARE THE BENEFITS OF ESSENTIAL OILS?

Aromatherapy is best for your brain because that's where your emotions are housed. Essential oils can get into your brain to help with many areas of health. I recommend stopping taking pills such as Advil and Aleve and try a different natural approach with Thyme, Rose, Clove or Eucalyptus anti-inflammatory oils. When energy and focus are the issues, try using citrus oils. The wild orange is a crowd pleaser and helps you focus on what you are doing, being present and eliminating distractions. The peppermint oil peps you up, gives you energy and can be mixed with water as a refreshing mouthwash. Refer to your vendor for dosage recommendation and note the quality oils such as DoTerra are a stronger pure form (no chemicals or pesticides sprayed on the source) and that grocery store brands are less potent.

WHERE TO PUT THE OILS?

Doterra recommends that you put oils on your chest and your wrist (wild orange and peppermint). Another essential oil blend is called True Blue rub. Add frankincense to create an amazing result for recovery on muscles. Lemon Grass is good for relieving muscle pain. You can put oils on the bottom of your feet at the reflexology points. Sandalwood oil is good for shutting the mind down and helping you sleep at night.

I found this quote that expresses much of what my personal journey is:

LIFE. Life is not a race - but indeed a journey. Be honest. Work hard. Be choosy. Say thank you, I love you, and great job to someone each day. Go to church. Take time for prayer. The Lord giveth and the Lord taketh. Let your handshake mean more than pen and paper. Love your life and what you've been given, it is not accidental - search for your purpose and do it as best you can. Dreaming does matter. It allows you to become that which you aspire to be. Laugh often. Appreciate the little things in life and enjoy them. Some of the best things really are free. Do not worry, less wrinkles are more becoming. Forgive, it frees the soul. Take time for yourself - plan for longevity. Recognize the special people you've been blessed to know. Live for today. Enjoy the moment. [Bonnie L. Mohr]

Get started on making small shifts in your life today by being more mindful and respectful of yourself. Mindfulness is the art of living in the present moment instead of going through life on auto-pilot. Make a decision to be more present and focused each day. Live in the present and start to become aware of your thoughts. You may be surprised to discover you are happier, more relaxed, and at peace from the inside out. If you are feeling stressed and anxious then try some of these tips to become more mindful, focused, and present, free of worry and expectations.

1. Mindful walking - practice daily
   a. Rhythm - align walking to the rhythm of your breath
   b. Be aware - how does the ground feel under your feet? What do you smell, hear and taste?
2. Mindful breathing - be aware of your breath and notice its ebb-and-flow while being in the present moment to cultivate a sense of calmness and peaceful mind.
   a. Get comfortable - be in a relaxed position.

      b.   Observe your breath - notice the coming and going of your breath

      c.   Be non-critical - focus the mind on the breath without being critical of self. Bring your attention back to the breath whenever you get distracted and mind wanders

3. Mindful eating - tune into the act of nourishment and create appreciate the food and environment around you at this moment

      a.   Take stock - what are your eating habits now?

      b.   Organization - focus on being present and not working as you eat or watching television.

      c.   Be sensitive - notice the feel of the food texture, the smells, and appearance.

4. Mindful Attitude - a skill that takes time but leads to a balance of awareness and serenity.

      a.   Non-judgment - learn how to non-judge everything and everyone.

      b.   Patience - practice the art of being in the moment daily.

      c.   Non-striving – don't set yourself up for disappointment and dissatisfaction instead doesn't have any expectation or purpose of being mindful.

      d.   Letting go - try not to cling on and get stuck to an experience that fills the mind up with clutter.

5. Focus on what you are doing now. When you get distracted and see a squirrel, bring your attention back to the one thing you are focused on. I am the queen of multi-tasking, but I am learning how to focus on one thing. Get in the zone and become more mindful. What can you do to become more calm and relaxed? I found I must eliminate distractions as on my cell phone and computer. Turn off the notifications and the access web pages open.

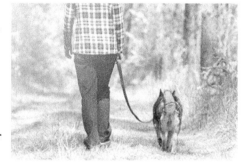

6. Join me in mastering the art of quieting the mind and pushing pauses occasionally.

7. Keep in mind that less is more. The more we do, the more risk of creating toxicity. Make sure you are being more mindful and putting more deposits into your wellness bank account. Find that delicate balance between doing too much and doing too little.

Let's start the transformation of taking a stroll through each day instead of racing through it. It is my deep desire that you need not pay the consequences as I did.

The big five WHOLESTIC Method Stress tips for becoming a fat burner:

1. _____
2. _____
3. _____
4. _____
5. _____

The WHOLESTIC Method to improving fat loss, health and performance for life and sports by working from the inside out.

ELEMENT #5
MOVEMENT

Does how much you move during the day make more of an impact on your ability to burn fat over how much you exercise each day?

Let's dive in... moving throughout the day is probably just as important as your morning thirty-minute workout session.

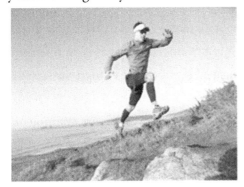

How long do you stay seated during the day? Did you know the average person spends nine to ten hours of their day *sitting*? Research shows that even if you work out every day, you cannot counteract the accumulated effects of continuous sitting for multiple hours a day. In fact, some say sitting is the new smoking.

The founder of medicine, Hippocrates, was a Greek physician who wrote the Hippocratic Oath 2,500 years ago:

Parts of the body, if they are unused and left idle, become liable to disease, defective in growth and age quickly.

According to the World Health Organization, "all parts of the body, if used in moderation and exercised in labors to which each is accustomed, become thereby healthy and well developed and age slowly; but if they are unused and left idle, they become liable to disease, defective in growth and age quickly." As the age of desk jobs matures, physical *inactivity* has risen to the fourth-leading risk factor for global mortality.

Yes, you heard that right. Desk jobs, be it on computers, telephones, or other machines are contributing to a serious world health issue. Those who drive all day are also at risk. Globally, six percent (6%) of deaths are attributed to physical **inactivity**. This follows high blood pressure (thirteen percent (13%)), tobacco use (nine percent (9%)) and is tied with deaths due high blood glucose (six percent (6%)). Moreover, physical inactivity is the main cause for approximately twenty-one to twenty-five percent (21-25%) of breast and colon cancers, twenty-seven percent (27%) of diabetes, and thirty percent (30%) of ischemic heart disease burden.

MAYO CLINIC STUDIES ON SITTING

The Mayo Clinic has done many studies on the effect of sitting too much. One study compared adults who spent less than two hours a day in front of the TV or other screen-based entertainment with those who logged more than four hours a day of recreational screen time.

Those with greater screen time had:

- A nearly fifty percent (50%) increased risk of death from any cause
- About a one hundred twenty-five percent (125%) increased risk of events associated with cardiovascular diseases, such as chest pain (angina) or heart attack

This increased risk was separate from other traditional risk factors for cardiovascular disease such as smoking or high blood pressure. They also note that any prolonged sitting is harmful even if one is spending a few hours a week at the gym or otherwise engaged in moderate or vigorous activity. This activity does not seem to offset the risk.

Think about it. We sit for work, transportation, television, and more. We are training and eating well (hopefully), but we could still be sitting ten to eleven hours or more per day. We could be sedentary for seventy percent (70%) of the day; the average person sits/lies/stationary twenty-three of twenty-four hours per day if you include sleeping, driving, eating, working, and watching social media/television. If you wake up and workout thirty to fifty minutes and then head to the office the rest of the day, we're all sitting too many hours of the day.

In order to mitigate the risks of sitting too much, the Mayo Clinic makes a few recommendations:

- Stand while talking on the phone or eating lunch.
- If you work at a desk for long periods of time, try a standing desk — or improvise with a high table or counter.
- Walk laps with your colleagues rather than gathering in a conference room for meetings.
- Position your work surface above a treadmill — with a computer screen and keyboard on a stand or a specialized treadmill-ready vertical desk — so that you can be in motion throughout the day.

I want you to improve your health by adding more movement to each and every day. This could be as simple as standing up for a minute or so each hour during the day. And yes, that is a weight loss tip: MOVE or at least STAND every hour. It sounds so simple, but we don't do it. Activity trackers such as Fitbit have reminders to get you up each hour. If that is not in the stars for you, set a timer to get up every hour during the workday.

In addition to the Mayo Clinic advice, I have a few more recommendations:

- Create a stand-up workstation. Then, alternate hours spent standing and sitting during the day.
- Take your 1:1s as walking meetings or move small group meetings to stand-up huddles and have water cooler meetings.
- Start wearing a tracking device to remind you to get up each hour.
  - Track how many steps you take per day. Strive to take at least 10,000 steps per day (though don't beat yourself up if you don't).
- Start drinking more water or tea so you get up to refill your water bottle as well as go to the bathroom. This keeps you hydrated as well.
- Improve your posture by standing up each hour for a chest opener stretch (interlace hands behind your back and lift away) or use the corner or door in your office to open your chest.
- Park at the back of the parking lot.
- Take the stairs if you are not on the ground floor.
- When at home watching TV, sit on the ground. You will find yourself leaning and shifting different positions when we sit on the floor.

SITTING IS THE NEW SMOKING

Scott Olsen and I recorded a *The WHOLE Athlete* podcast episode about "Sitting is the new Smoking." Too much sitting every day is resulting in health issues that are reinforcing the importance of regular movement in the fitness industry. Movement training and teaching the proper mechanics of everyday movement patterns is going mainstream. Scott (www.beyondthemuscle.com) is an accomplished bodyworker and physical therapist who specializes in manual therapy to help his clients reduce chronic pain including joint pain around tendons and muscles. He teaches movement drills to biomechanically hold their joints and body structure in place for life movements each day.

From my experience in the fitness industry, there is a slow increase in awareness of recovery for training athletes of all levels. I believe in heart rate training to exercise the aerobic engine (MAFF heart rate aerobic zone), interspersed with recovery movement days. Remember, training hard every day does not allow the body to recover and does not compensate for sitting the rest of the day. Recovery days (use HRV to determine your recovery) provide a great opportunity to get in the habit of moving each how throughout the day.

WHY SITTING IS HARMFUL

While many of us have been nagged by our mothers to sit up straight, people don't do it. In addition, most people have never been taught how to move with correct posture. This is what happens if we are disconnected from our own bodies.

When we are sitting down in a comfortable chair, we don't stay engaged in our deep postural muscles. When you sit in your favorite chair or spot to watch TV, your body tends to become molded to the sofa cushion in the same position you are sitting in. Then when you get up to move and participate in basic life movements, your basic movement mechanics suffer. Why is this?

Some muscles get longer/lengthened and some muscles get shortened or tight. Too much sitting results in tight, shortened hamstrings, the adductors let go, shortened hip flexors, rounding of the back, and a compressed the belly. All our basic human movement patterns have become turned off so we could efficiently sit in our favorite seat or position on the sofa. I don't know about you but I don't want to be walking around looking like my sofa. Scott learned from his chronic back pain to sit in an uncomfortable, wooden chair. He would start to sit more upright as he was less comfortable. You can modify your environment by setting up less comfortable options like Scott did.

When we sit on our booty most of the day we are compressing skin, lymphatic fluid, fascia, muscles, fat, and other necessary layers of our body. When we take any parts of our body and compress it for too long, we will have trouble and dysfunction as limited blood flow and cells start to adapt to this chronic sitting patterns. Prolonged sitting will turn off muscles and we can run higher risks of cancer and Type 2 diabetes.

We need a stimulation of varied environmental conditions: the room, the temperature, and the movement patterns that change the shape of the body instead of encouraging the same movement patterns repeatedly. As I say often to clients, muscle confusion is ideal for workouts, and greasing the groove throughout the day is a wonderful way to enhance this. Our hips are becoming tight and our spinal alignment is becoming more forward flexion. It's no wonder that hip replacement surgery is becoming commonplace amongst relatively young people.

When Scott Olsen works with clients who have complicated pain patterns, he looks at stagnation or flow. Much of this stagnation is due to compression of joints, tendons, fascia and blood vessels. If we have a compressed joint, it won't feel good. If we have a compressed tendon, it doesn't feel good. The goal should be more to add more space in our body by stretching, moving and varying our position. Yoga is an excellent way to open and stretch all the joints.

LEARNING HOW TO MOVE

Now that we know that we need to move more throughout the day, it is time to discuss how we move as this can have a profound effect on our health in terms of staying injury and pain-free.

Most people yank their bodies around with no thought or awareness of how they are moving. The thing is that we can learn to create a deeper engagement with our movement, especially by engaging our hips, thighs, and core. By pushing more into the ground and using our feet to help fire the correct muscles to stay upright we train ourselves to move in a safe and strengthening way. Most people sit up by pulling themselves forward with the head, shoulders, and spine instead of using the core muscles. Next time you sit up in bed pay attention. Did you engage your core? I am teaching people how to move better and engage the glutes by pushing or driving more into the lead leg. Feel your glutes and learn how to activate the correct muscles. Avoid glute amnesia by creating glute muscle memory.

Another common movement faux pas is to drag yourself up a staircase using your head and neck. A good habit to acquire is to pause at the top or bottom of stairs, lift your shoulders up, back and then down, engage your core, then proceed. You will find yourself going up and down stairs with your head held high in no time at all, while at the same time strengthening your core and proper posture muscles for use in other movements.

Scott suggests walking around holding a medicine ball or kettlebell so that you will become more alert as you are walking and learn to turn on the postural muscles. After that go sit with the weight and feel the structure of the body change with your increased awareness of postural muscles.

We need to be strong enough to go from lying on the floor to standing up without using your neck and back to pull ourselves up. That said most people have lost healthy structure and strength to move correctly and activate the correct muscles and movement patterns. I started training clients how to move from the ground to standing based on observing people's movement patterns. I throw some cards on the floor and teach clients how to pick them up with proper form. You too can learn to engage the proper muscles and move with proper posture and strength.

Start small by creating new habits. It will take time, so pick one goal at a time to implement into your daily schedule. Find the minimum effective dose that doesn't feel too challenging and have some fun creating new habits and muscle memories. Stick with it for long-term. If sitting is the new smoking, then it may be a hard habit to quit, but you can do it. Standing is better than sitting, but inactivity is the issue. Shift, move, sway and take breaks. Don't stay still for too long.

For more information on Scott Olsen, visit www.beyondthemuscle.com.

MOVEMENT AND WORKOUT TIPS:

1. Plan workout schedule for the week ahead. Remember your goal is to MOVE thirty minutes per day and 10,000 steps per day. Wear your heart rate monitor for workouts.
2. Schedule in two to three strength training with some higher intensity interval workouts fifteen to thirty minutes each week.
3. Purchase a FITBIT or other tracker to monitor SLEEP and MOVEMENT.
   a. Sleep (Goal 7-9 hours per night)
   b. Daily steps (Goal 10,000 per day)
   c. Idle Time (Move every hour)
   d. Hourly steps (Goal 250 steps/hour)
   e. Estimated Calories burned (500 calories above basal metabolic rate)
4. Add rest and restore exercise sessions as nature walks and yoga.

The big five WHOLESTIC Method Movement tips for becoming a fat burner:
1. _____
2. _____
3. _____
4. _____
5. _____

The WHOLESTIC Method to improving fat loss, health and performance for life and sports by working from the inside out.

REFERENCES:

Huffington Post - http://tinyurl.com/SittingNewSmoking

Runners World - http://tinyurl.com/SittingNewSmoking1

Forbes - http://tinyurl.com/SittingNewSmoking2

ELEMENT #6
DIGESTION, GUT HEALTH, AND HORMONE BALANCE

Digestion and Gut Health is a major topic and is challenging to limit to one chapter, however, I'll give you an overview of how important digestion, gut health, and hormone balance is to our ability to burn fat as well as feel and move better.

In recent years the gut has been referred to as the second brain and the link between the nervous system and the digestive system has been recognized and studied. Some refer to this link as a third, *Enteric* branch of the Autonomic Nervous System. Most people have experienced the 'butterflies" in the stomach before an important event or during stressful times. This illustrates the link between our emotions, state of mind and our gut.

In addition, the microbiome (our gut bacteria) has received a lot of attention in many medical and wellness circles. The microbiome has been implicated in a wide range of conditions from inflammatory bowel diseases to asthma and according to the Human Microbiome Project, the gut microbiome even influences our circadian rhythms.

Another new kid on the block is leaky gut syndrome. Leaky gut is a condition that occurs when the layer of cells lining the intestinal wall become irritated. Normally these cells absorb particles from food (or toxins or edible food-like substances) though if the cells get damaged they can become porous or leaky, allowing food and other particles to "leak" out of the gut and into the bloodstream. Not good.

Unbeknownst to many, our hormones are tied to the health of our guts and vice versa. For example, when you have hypothyroidism it's easy to get caught up in the thyroid lab results and meds. While these are significant, it is also (maybe more) important to remember that gut health is the foundation of thyroid health and that as long as you struggle with a leaky gut or other digestive issues, you will never experience optimum thyroid health.

Let's work our way through the wondrous world of the gut, starting with good 'ole digestion.

DIGESTION BASICS

Where do you think digestion begins? The stomach? The mouth? Actually, digestion begins in the brain. The sight and smell of food activates the salivary glands to start producing saliva. Who knew?

The tenth cranial nerve we met in previous chapters, also known as the vagus nerve, communicates with the stomach and the pancreas. When the signal is sent, the stomach starts producing hydrochloric acid (HCL) and the pancreas starts producing insulin and is prepped to produce digestive enzymes. The vagus nerve also signals the gallbladder when it needs to contract and to start releasing bile and it tells the small intestine to start producing hormones for digestion. As you may recall, the vagus nerve is part of the parasympathetic nervous system which is also known as the "rest and digest" branch of the autonomic nervous system and so it is advantageous to rest while we digest.

Carbohydrates generally digest faster than protein and fats and protein digests faster than fats, so the mechanism for each varies.

CARBOHYDRATE DIGESTION

Carbohydrate digestion begins in the mouth as enzymes in the saliva, called *Salivary Amylase* and the mechanical act of chewing start to break them down even before they reach the stomach. If we don't start to break down the starch in the mouth, then digestion will be impacted (can you say indigestion?) Once the food is chewed and broken down by the saliva, it is now called bolus and is swallowed. While carb breakdown continues in the stomach, most, with the exception of alcohol, are absorbed in the small intestine. Cells lining the small intestine secrete enzymes which break complex carbs into simple sugars so the body can then absorb.

There are several types of carbs, depending on the number of chemical bonds they contain. Simple sugars contain just one or two bonds while complex carbs must be split into simple sugars before they can be absorbed. Fruits are an example of simple sugars while vegetables and whole grains represent complex carbs. Fiber is a type of carbohydrate that usually can't be used for energy. It remains intact until it reaches the large intestine where a small amount is broken down by bacteria and absorbed.

PROTEIN DIGESTION

Protein digestion occurs mostly in the stomach. Upon swallowing, the food (now called bolus) reaches the stomach and the hormone Gastrin is released to stimulate the gastric glands for the release of pepsinogen (an inactive form of pepsin) and hydrochloric acid (HCL) to uncoil the protein strands and break them down. Trypsin, another enzyme, breaks the protein strands into molecules containing one, two or three amino acids in the small intestine, where nearly all the protein is digested. Any remaining will pass through the large intestine.

FAT DIGESTION

Although fats stay in your stomach the longest, very little fat digestion occurs in the stomach. Bile from the liver prepares fat for breakdown by emulsifying it, making it water soluble. This makes it easier for enzymes to break the fat into smaller pieces for digestion. In the small intestine, the pancreatic enzyme lipase splits the fats into fatty acid and glycerol which are then absorbed by the body.

Want more hairy details? Here we go.

When the bolus becomes chyme in the stomach, the food (now chyme) moves into the start of the small intestine, the duodenum, where lots of digestion steps occur.

- In the small intestine, the hormones Secretin and CCK (cholecystokinin) are released in small amounts.
- The pancreas will receive a message from the hormone CCK from the first part of the small intestine—the duodenum—to stimulate the release of digestive enzymes.
- The hormone CCK will stimulate emptying the bile (required for fat digestion) from the gallbladder (storage unit for bile made in the liver).
- The hormone Secretin is released in the duodenum as well to signal the secretion of sodium bicarbonate from the pancreas to raise the pH levels in the small intestine (stomach is highly acidic to break down food—bolus—into chyme and more processes).
- The release of Secretin in the small intestine—duodenum—also stimulates the digestion

of fat by secreting bile in the gallbladder to the liver into the duodenum.

When the chyme enters the small intestine (duodenum) pancreatic amylase is released to digest the carbohydrates (polysaccharides into disaccharides into monosaccharides). Brush border enzymes, found on the tiny hair-like projections called microvilli, are released from the lining and complete the breakdown of the disaccharides into forms of glucose. (Enzymes such as: fructose, fructose, Maltase maltose, lactase, lactose). Once the nutrients are absorbed into the bloodstream, any remains from the carbohydrate digestion get passed into the large intestine and turned into the feces.

MICROBIOME

The body's microbiome consists of colonies of various microbes that reside in your gut and elsewhere in your body. It is unique to each person and can be quickly altered based on diet, lifestyle, exposure to toxins and antibiotics. According to Dr. Mercola, there are approximate 1,000 species of bacteria living you your body and they outnumber the number of cells 10 to 1. In addition, he says that you also harbor viruses which outnumber bacteria 10 to 1. These 100 trillion bacteria and quadrillion viruses perform a multitude of functions and need to be properly balanced and cared for in order to maintain good health. None of these are good or bad unless potentially harmful ones start to outnumber the others. This is being germ-phobic is not good. Health-promoting bacteria can be killed when we use anti-bacterial soaps, hand sanitizers, and antibiotics.

We have a symbiotic relationship with our microbiome and keeping it in balance and healthy is just as important as getting enough exercise and sleep. A healthy microbiome boosts our immune system, keeps your gut lining healthy and is implicated in the inflammatory response. When they are out of balance it can make you weak, tired and inflamed. This gut bacteria produces nutrients, as well as help you absorb nutrients. Most of the Vitamin K made in your body each day comes from this bacteria, and since your body does not store Vitamin K well; it is crucial that your gut production is in order. The microbiome also heavily influences your B vitamins and helps you make and absorb Vitamin B12.

As I mentioned, the gut is connected to the ANS via the Enteric branch. Relatively recent research has found that the *Gut-Brain Axis* consists of bidirectional communication between the central and enteric nervous system, linking emotional and cognitive centers of the brain with peripheral intestinal functions. There is clinical evidence that links microbial imbalance is linked to central nervous disorders such as autism, anxiety, and depression, as well as gastrointestinal disorders like Irritable Bowel Syndrome (IBS and leaky gut syndrome.

https://www.ncbi.nlm.nih.gov/pmc/articles/PMC4367209

LEAKY GUT

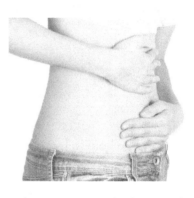

How often do you eat foods resulting in a bloated belly, gas, or a headache? You could be suffering from a leaky gut. Leaky gut is just what it says, a condition where holes develop in the walls of the gut allowing intestinal contents to leak out into the bloodstream. This includes undigested proteins that can trigger allergies or autoimmune disease as well as bacteria that do not belong in your bloodstream. Once they leak out they can impact your internal organs causing inflammation and leading to disease.

Our dependence on fast and processed foods is wreaking havoc in our bodies as the prepared, manufactured, man-made, fake foods have become a staple in our society. If you haven't already heard it's called SAD, the Standard American Diet. Gotta love the irony of that name. The SAD diet and western lifestyle are leading to a lower diversity of bacteria in the gut, opening the door for a leaky gut. The root cause of most of our auto-immune disorders seems to be a result of a leaky gut which is a cause of a lot more as we will touch upon.

Symptoms of a Leaky Gut

A leaky gut can lead to inflammation throughout your system and can cause symptoms, such as:

- Bloating
- Food sensitivities
- Thyroid conditions
- Fatigue
- Joint pain
- Headaches
- Skin issues like rosacea and acne
- Digestive problems

- Weight gain
- Syndrome X

What causes a leaky gut?

- A diet low in probiotics
- A diet high in sugar and processed foods
- A diet high in grains and conventional dairy (especially cow's milk)
- Overuse of medications including NSAIDs, antibiotics, aspirin, hormones as birth control
- Bacterial imbalances
- High emotional stress is a major cause of diseases, especially digestive ones
- Hormone imbalances – cortisol high to cause yeast to grow
- Overuse of antibiotics and underuse of probiotics

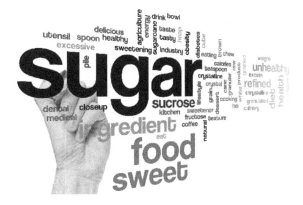
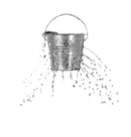

All I think about when I hear the word leaky gut is the song...

There's a hole in the bucket, dear Liza, dear Liza.
There's a hole in the bucket, dear Liza. There's a hole.

DIGESTION, THE GUT, AND THE ENDOCRINE SYSTEM

The digestive and endocrine systems work together, mostly through the pancreas, to produce and disseminate the digestive enzymes. The endocrine system consists of the hypothalamus, pituitary, parathyroid, adrenal glands, reproductive glands, thyroid, and pineal gland. The primary role of this system is to produce hormones that signal the digestive system to start and stop. Most all digestive disorders are related to auto-immune and inflammatory disease which is related to an inflamed gut which leads to leaky gut which then leads to inflammation in the body and so on in a vicious circle.

A major symptom of my burnout included elevated cortisol, so let's talk about the impact of chronically elevated cortisol and how it disrupts Endocrine System balance leading to the dreaded Endocrine Cascade. If one hormone is overly depended upon, it becomes worn out or exhausted and we are at risk of creating a hormonal cascade or a domino effect in the hormonal system (endocrine system). Our endocrine system is like an orchestra; the band must work altogether.

There are multiple ways where chronically elevated cortisol disrupts Endocrine System balance including:

- Low T3 (Thyroid)
- Low DHEA
- Low Progesterone
- Pituitary Imbalance
- Estrogen Dominance
- Androgen Dominance
- Thyroid Metabolism

The result of too much cortisol will require the pancreas to release more insulin as the liver is making more glucose to keep up with the demand (as a response from the increased cortisol). The insulin receptors on the cells get exhausted as they have to keep knocking on the cells to ask for entry to uptake the excess blood glucose levels. Eventually, the cell receptors don't respond fast enough resulting in overworking the pancreas.

Then, we get insulin resistance from the elevated cortisol levels which lead to more problems:

- Poor mineral absorption by cells
- Inflammation issues - excess insulin blocks our Prostaglandin One pathway
- Elevated blood pressure and cholesterol
- Increased estrogen levels in men
- Increased testosterone level in women

We need to remember that the body is all connected and we need to treat it as a WHOLE system. If the adrenal glands are constantly activated from various forms of stress, then we are continuously stimulating the Hypothalamus to tell the pituitary gland to notify the adrenal gland to release the hormone cortisol to deal with the perceived threat. Anytime we activate or do anything too often or too frequently we increase the risk of breaking something. This includes or overuses injury which also leads to dysfunction. That dysfunction doesn't only impact the adrenal glands but the entire endocrine system as it all works together.

Thyroid problems seem to be the medical issue de jour. And yes, your thyroid gland plays a big role in your digestion. Though guess what, it goes the other way around as well. Gut health can actually influence the health of the thyroid (and entire endocrine system). This makes complete sense given what we have talked about here. The SAD has ruined the microbiome, which has caused leaky guts and affected the endocrine system. The thyroid may be particularly susceptible to leaky gut complications. According to Dr. Josh Axe, "to heal any condition, including thyroid, hormones, brain, or joints, you must heal your gut first."

Dr. Amy Myers of the Thyroid Connection and The Auto-Immune Solution shares on her blog:

Gluten is one of the main causes of leaky gut in people that I see with thyroid issues and autoimmune diseases, and not just among celiac patients, but for anyone with gluten sensitivity. When anyone, whether they have gluten sensitivity or not, eats a gluten-containing food, the gluten proteins make their way through the stomach and arrive at the small intestine, where the body responds by producing zonulin, a chemical that signals the tight junctions of the intestinal walls to open up, creating temporary permeability. This permeability will heal as the gut cells renew every forty-eight hours. ... you have gluten sensitivity and eat gluten, then this permeability will not heal in that forty-eight hours and your gut remains leaky. Leaky gut can also be caused or exacerbated by gut infections such as Candida overgrowth or SIBO... antibiotics, steroids, or birth control pills, as well as a high-stress lifestyle. New research shows spraying... (Roundup) on... wheat is... a major contributor of leaky gut and gluten sensitivity.

I asked Dr. Amy Myers, the author of The Thyroid Connection about the thyroid connection to our health and digestion. Dr. Myers recently wrote a blog that caught my eye *Is Gluten to Blame for Your Thyroid Dysfunction?*

In Dr. Myer's first book, *The Autoimmune Solution,* she explains the hazards of gluten for those with autoimmunity and how gluten is also damaging and inflammatory to the thyroid. She explains what thyroid dysfunction, hypothyroidism, and hyperthyroidism are in *The Thyroid Connection.* The important thing to know is most autoimmunity causes thyroid dysfunction. Autoimmune disorders are when your immune system mistakenly attacks your own tissues. In the case of thyroid dysfunction, this attack can cause the thyroid to underproduce – (Hashimoto's Disease) or over produce thyroid hormones (Graves' disease).

Gluten plays a very important role in this because it not only triggers high inflammation, which stresses your immune system and eventually causes it to attack your own tissues, it also looks very chemically similar to your thyroid, which causes something called molecular mimicry. Molecular mimicry is when your body mistakes one substance (in this case your thyroid tissues) for something else (gluten) because they look so similar. This means when you eat gluten foods, your body mounts a defense against the gluten, but also attacks your thyroid by mistake.

Dr. Myers suggests getting thyroid panel breakdown to see the whole picture. Read more in her new book, *The Thyroid Connection.*

She included the ranges for each marker she has found to be optimal for both herself and her patients:

- TSH 1-2 UIU/ML or lower
- Free T4 >1. 1 NG/DL
- Free T3 > 3. 2 PG/ML
- Reverse T3 > 10:1 ratio RT3:FT3
- Thyroid Peroxidase Antibodies < 4 IU/ML or negative
- Thyroglobulin Antibodies < 4 IU/ML or negative

Dr. Myers explores how gluten can create chaos in your gut, increase your inflammation and cause your immune system to attack your own thyroid. As we continue to learn, gluten is one of the main causes of leaky gut, and most people are unaware of this as their symptoms become normal functions to them over time.

A quick note on gluten and why the recent gluten sensitivity craze. The wheat we eat today is not the wheat your grandmother ate. It is a hybridized variety that is designed for high yield. In addition, many farmers spray the wheat with the poison Roundup to make harvesting easier. So not only are you eating wheat that is not particularly friendly, it is made poisonous with the glyphosate from Roundup. I recommend reading "Wheat Belly: Lose the Wheat, Lose the Weight and Find Your Path Back to Health by William Davis MD. It is an easy and valuable read.

FOOD INTOLERANCES

Which came first, the chicken or the egg? This is the question when examining the link between leaky gut and food intolerances. Most of us have some sort of food intolerance, meaning that while we are not full over allergic, our body has a low-level reaction and is often unable to fully digest some foods. These partially broken down foods can actually attack the lining of the small intestine, creating tiny holes in the tissue. This compromises the gut's ability to absorb nutrients and filter toxins. Malabsorption can lead to vitamin deficiencies, anemia, and osteoporosis while filtration failure can lead to a host of autoimmune diseases such as rheumatoid arthritis, colitis, eczema, Celiac and Crohn's, not to mention hormonal disruption and infection vulnerability

On the other side of the coin, gut issues will, over time, create food intolerances and food issues. Many people are unaware they are sensitive to food such as eggs, peanuts, tree nuts, and/or dairy. These food intolerances are displayed in the body and are a warning sign of a leaky gut. I strongly suggest learning more about leaky gut, digestive disorders, food sensitivities, and ADHD type of disorders if you have any of these warning signs and abnormalities, as the symptoms can be improved by improving your diet, your digestion system, and healing your gut.

Because it is a vicious cycle, it is important to identify food sensitivities and eliminate these foods from your diet as you repair your gut. Fortunately, there is a free app by SweetWater Health, called FoodEffect, which can help you detect these low-level sensitivities. For Android, the same app is available on Google Play and is called Bulletproof Food Detective. Learn more at www.SweetWaterHRV.com.

HORMONE IMBALANCE

Many men and women suffer from hormone imbalances as a result of poor digestion. We need to focus on strengthening and improving our digestion, blood sugar handling, essential fatty acids, minerals, and hydration, then, continue to evaluate symptoms and investigate the root cause. Rather than taking hormone supplements each day, we need to determine what is out of balance. I found out my stomach HCL wasn't correct (not low enough) and my liver wasn't functioning as well – plus my essential fatty acids and minerals were low. By building up our foundation based on facts rather than conjecture, we can make progress naturally using the body's own innate intelligence.

Fat Loss Hormones:

Now let's look some of your key hormones that play into fat loss. Leptin and ghrelin are primary in the regulation of food intake and body weight in humans.

Leptin and ghrelin are two hormones that have been recognized to have a major influence on energy balance. They are referred to as the hunger hormones: leptin, and ghrelin. Leptin is a hormone, made by fat cells, that decreases your appetite. Ghrelin is a hormone that increases appetite and plays a role in body weight.

- **Leptin** is a mediator of long-term regulation of energy balance, suppressing food intake and thereby inducing weight loss.
- **Ghrelin,** on the other hand, is a fast-acting hormone, seemingly playing a role in meal initiation.

As a growing number of people suffer from obesity, understanding the mechanisms by which various hormones and neurotransmitters have an influence on energy balance has been a subject of intensive research. In obese subjects, the circulating level of the anorexigenic hormone **leptin is increased**, whereas surprisingly, the level of the orexigenic **hormone ghrelin is decreased**. It is now established that obese patients are **leptin-resistant**. However, the way both the leptin and ghrelin systems contribute to the development or maintenance of obesity is yet not clear. The purpose of this review is to provide background information on the leptin and ghrelin hormones, their role in food intake and body weight in humans, and their mechanism of action. Possible abnormalities in the leptin and ghrelin systems that may contribute to the development of obesity will be mentioned. In addition, the potentials of leptin and ghrelin as drug targets will be discussed. Finally, the influence of the diet on leptin and ghrelin secretion and functioning will be described.

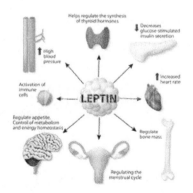

Ghrelin

- Ghrelin is your hunger gremlin.
- It is produced in your stomach and, like many fat-loss hormones works with your brain to signal that you are hungry.

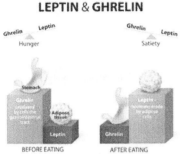

LEPTIN & GHRELIN

- Reducing calories, to lose weight, causes an increase in ghrelin.
- Even after twelve months of a reduced-calorie diet, research shows that ghrelin levels stay elevated. In other words, your body never adapts to eating less and constantly sends the "I'm hungry" signal, which is why maintaining weight loss is often harder than losing it first.
- The good news: Intense exercise decreases ghrelin levels, making it a key component to fat loss and weight maintenance.

Leptin

- Leptin is a type of hormone called an adipokine that is released exclusively from fat cells.
- Leptin interacts with your brain to get your body to eat less and burn more calories.
- The more body fat you have, the more Leptin your fat cells will release.
- Too much body fat leads to too much Leptin being released, a condition called Leptin resistance.
- With Leptin Resistance, your brain becomes numb to leptin's signal.
- To maximize Leptin sensitivity, get adequate sleep and pack your diet full of antioxidant-rich berries and green and red vegetables.
- Losing weight also enhances Leptin sensitivity and gives you momentum, as the more weight you lose, the more effective Leptin will become in your body.

Adiponectin

- Adiponectin is another adipokine, but unlike Leptin, the leaner your body is the more adiponectin your fat cells will release.
- Adiponectin enhances your muscle's ability to use carbohydrates for energy, boosts your metabolism, increase the rate in which your body breaks down fat, and curbs your appetite.
- You can maximize your adiponectin levels by moving more during the day (getting leaner) and replacing carbohydrates in your diet with monounsaturated fats (olives, avocados, etc.)

Insulin

- Insulin plays a very important role in your body and is key for recovering from exercise, muscle building, and maintaining optimal blood sugar levels.
- When carbohydrate intakes are high and insulin is left to run wild in the body, it can inhibit the breakdown and burning of stored fat. Insulin and carbohydrates are very tightly linked.
- The more carbohydrates you eat; the more insulin will be released.
- To optimize insulin for fat loss, aim to get most of your carbohydrates from vegetables and some fruit. Limit grains and starches to smaller portions directly after exercise.

Glucagon

- Glucagon is a hormone that acts directly opposite to insulin.
- While insulin stores carbohydrates and builds fat, glucagon is responsible for breaking down stored carbohydrates and fats and releasing them so your body can use them for energy.
- Eating a protein-rich, low carbohydrate meal is the best way to maximize glucagon release.

CCK

- Short for Cholecystokinin, this hormone is released from the cells in your intestines whenever you eat protein or fat.
- CCK doesn't just stay in your gut. Instead, it communicates with your nervous system to flip the satiety switch while simultaneously working with your stomach to slow the rate of digestion.
- The result is that you feel fuller longer. Take full advantage of CCK by making sure you have protein and fat at every meal.

Epinephrine

- Known as a fight or flight hormone, epinephrine drives the burning of fat and its release for energy in the body.
- Epinephrine can also aid in appetite suppression.
- Exercise is the best way to turn on epinephrine release in your body, interval training cranks up epinephrine.

Growth Hormone

- Considered to be the fountain of youth by many, growth hormone also helps with fat loss.
- Growth hormone interacts with fat cells and coaxes them to break down and burn stored fat for energy.

- Growth hormone can be increased through an intense exercise like intervals or circuit training and sleep.

As you can see there are so many hormones that are affected by your digestive health and most of these hormones contribute directly to your ability to burn fat and keep the hunger down and weight off. Moving forward, the key is to fix an unhealthy gut and then maintain that health.

RESTORING YOUR DIGESTIVE AND HORMONAL HEALTH

Digestive health is a key component for supporting most all systems in our body. Digestive disease is linked to some of the fastest growing diseases in our country today. Approximately 60 to 70 million people per year (and growing) are affected by digestive diseases. As we mentioned, the brain is a giant pattern matcher and filter and will remove from immediate awareness most conditions that are familiar even if they are dysfunctional. You may have a condition that feels normal to you is actually some form of digestive disease and so it is critical to find out if you have any food sensitivities or intolerances. If you do, remove those foods from your diet and then proceed with the process of restoring digestive health.

While the Food Effect app is free and easy, it does require you to enter your foods and take your pulse multiple times a day. If this feels like too much for you, I recommend you talk to Christopher Kelly, at www.nourishbalancethrive.com, for a complimentary consultation and to order lab tests. You won't know what is going on under the hood unless you do some investigating.

Unfortunately, many traditional allopathic doctors did not study nutrition or the microbiome in medical school and thus don't offer this functional lab test. Also, because it is so new, leaky gut syndrome (similar to adrenal fatigue) is not an official diagnosis and so you will need to seek out an MD that specializes in Functional or Naturopathic medicine, or visit a Chiropractor or other wellness professional to diagnosis the root cause of our health problems and imbalances.

As a side note, our allopathic western doctors are trained to treat disease, usually with a quick method such as a pill, a shot, or surgery rather than figuring out the root cause of the problem, ailment, or issue. Masking the symptoms or cutting out a piece of the body will not ultimately heal the underlying cause. This is true in so many areas in medicine.

Dr. Josh Axe suggests the top seven foods to heal leaky gut and the leaky gut diet. Consuming the foods listed below will help you improve your gut. We all want a healthy happy gut and a happy body.

Foods to heal gut: leaky gut diet

- Bone Broth (fast with bone broth, apple cider vinegar)
  - Bone broth is already broken down into amino acids
  - 8-ounce cup, twice each day
- Easily digestible carbs – vegetables, fruit, and raw honey
- Easily digested fats - Ghee, coconut oil, egg yolk
- Easily digested protein - wild caught salmon, grass-fed beef, and chicken
- Probiotic-Rich Foods such as sauerkraut, yogurt, kefir, and fermented foods
- Flax seeds
- In addition, eliminate processed grains and processed foods from your diet and focus on consuming these superfoods.

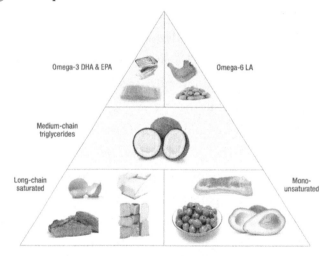

Supplements:

1. Digestive enzymes: two caps with meals to help break down proteins and fats
2. Probiotics: two caps, three times per day
3. L-Glutamine: protects the gut wall lining from different exposures
4. Healthy Fatty Acids: fermented cod liver oil, fish oil or krill oil. 1000mg daily
5. Peppermint essential oils can help the gut

Here are some tips on how to balance your hormones naturally:

Top foods to support thyroid health include selenium, iodine (only ten percent (10%) of hypothyroid), protein, probiotics, and omega 3s.

1. *Thyroid supporting foods*: Brazil nuts, wild caught salmon, seaweeds, organic protein sources and probiotic foods.

2. *Eat a variety of short, medium and long-chain* **essential fatty acids** as grass-fed butter, coconut oil, avocados, and wild salmon. These fats are required building blocks for hormone production, boost your metabolism and help with weight loss. Dr. Josh Axe recommends these five fats you must have to naturally balance your hormones:

    *   *Healthy Omega 9 Fats*: Avocadoes, Almonds, Olive Oil which are also monounsaturated fats. Add one serving to a meal each day.
    *   *Short Chain Fatty Acid* (Grass-fed Butter, grass-fed Ghee, organic Kefir, and organic full-fat yogurt to help gut health and aids in the production of B12 and K2 vitamins.
    *   *Omega 3 Fatty Acid:* Wild Caught Salmon, Chia seeds, Flax seeds, Walnuts which reduce inflammation in the body.
    *   *Medium Chain Fatty Acid:* Coconut oil and Coconut Products which the body can burn coconut oil as energy and help balance blood sugar levels. Too much sugar and not enough good fats imbalances our hormones as insulin.
    *   *GLA:* An omega-6 fat found in hemp seeds or evening primrose oil and borage oil. Try adding a tablespoon of hemp seeds in your morning shake.

3. *Balance the Omega 3/6 Intake:*

    *   We consume too much vegetable oils in our regular food plan which are Omega 6 fatty acids and can cause inflammation in the body which can contribute to chronic diseases.
    *   Strive for 1:1 Omega 6 to Omega 3 ratio rather than our current average 20:1
    *   Avoid oils high in omega-6 fatty acids: safflower, sunflower, corn, cottonseed, canola, soybean, and peanut oils.
    *   Add more omega-3 fatty acids: wild fish, flaxseed, chia seeds, walnuts, and grass-fed animal products.
    *   Add one type of omega-6 fatty acids that are beneficial: GLA (gamma-linoleic acid) in supplement form by using evening primrose oil or borage oil or find

in hemp seeds. Studies show supplementing with GLA can support healthy progesterone hormone levels.

4. ***Try adding Adaptogen supplements*** include Ashwagandha, holy basil, licorice root, Rhodiola, and ginseng. Adaptogen herbs are healing plants that help promote hormone balance, improve the immune system, support natural energy levels, combat stress and protect the body from various diseases.

   - *Licorice root*: Reducing stress, stress on GI system and emotional stress
   - *Ashwagandha and Holy Basil*: improve thyroid function, lower cholesterol, reduce brain cell degeneration, reducing anxiety, lower depression, stabilizing blood sugar and best of all support the adrenal glands.
   - *Rhodiola and Ginseng*: improves blood sugar, athletic performance, energy metabolism, fat loss, and brain function.

5. ***Heal your Gut:*** I believe that most of all us have some leaks in our gut wall lining from the food we have eaten over the years that we thought were healthy as well as from all the prescription medications and antibiotics we were given over the years when we were unaware of the side effects on our gut health. Any leaks, holes, or gaps in our gut wall lining (leaky gut) not only impacts our digestive system, but they create chaos in our hormonal system; specifically, our thyroid. Our internal health is a domino effect. It all starts in the gut or with any type of excessive stress.

Our gut wall lining and digestive system get damaged from:
- Processed foods
- Gluten
- Hydrogenated Oils
- Emotional Stress

Often, we have an imbalance in good and bad bacteria in our gut due to the leaky gut syndrome. We are adding ***probiotics and digestive enzyme supplements*** into our daily program to help improve and repair our gut health which can lead to improving our hormone balance.

www.fitnessforwardstudio.com/wholesticmethod

6. ***Eliminate Toxins***: Detox your household and environment including your kitchen, cleaning supplies and body care products. Switch from drinking out of plastic including plastic straws, BPA, Teflon, oxybenzone, triclosan, dioxins, and parabens are other toxins we need to reduce the use of daily. Remember not to freeze or heat your BPA plastic bottles and Teflon pans as you will increase the risk for toxins to leach out.

    - Recycle your plastic water and drinking bottles and replace with glass or stainless steel to reduce BPA toxic effects.
    - Trade out Switch from Teflon pans to stainless steel, ceramic or cast iron pans to help reduce toxins when cooking.
    - Eliminate conventional body care products and replace with natural non-toxic ingredients.
    - Products that we grew up with are high in DEA, parabens, propylene glycol and sodium lauryl sulfate. Check out your favorite household products on here http://www.ewg.org/skindeep/ to find out how they rank.

7. ***Exercise***: The right type of exercise and frequency can increase levels of endorphins, testosterone, and growth hormone, as well as help, regulate insulin levels and cortisol levels. HIIT training (cardioblasts) mixed with strength training or just strength training more effective than chronic cardio or endurance training for hormone balance, fat loss, and health:
    - Improve metabolism and immune system
    - Reduces depression (any form of exercise)
    - Supports thyroid hormone balance. High-Intensity Interval Training (HIIT)
    - Increases testosterone and DHEA (weight training and HIIT) and can even slow the aging process.
    - Endurance exercise increases cortisol levels (catabolic) where interval training and strength training (anabolic) can lower the cortisol levels as well as slow the aging process.
    - Avoid HIIT when fighting adrenal fatigue instead try lighter exercise as light strength training, yoga, Pilates, and Barre type of exercise.
    - Building muscle tissue helps balance blood sugar levels.

- Add quick cardio blasts into strength training sessions for 15-30 minutes total, 2-3 times per week maximum (more is not better.)

8. ***Sleep:*** Make sure you sleep seven to nine hours per night. If you get less than seven hours of sleep per night, it could weaken your immune system. See our sleep section for more on how to get more sleep.

9. ***Limit Caffeine Consumption:*** Excessive caffeine can be another stressor and lead to elevated cortisol levels, lowers thyroid hormone levels and contribute to a weakened immune system. Avoid stimulants as caffeine if you have any adrenal fatigue or thyroid issues. Try some green tea or herbal teas instead and go for a walk outside instead to wake up or do some jumping jacks.

10. ***Vitamin D3:*** Two roles...vitamin and a hormone that works with the immune system, emotional health, bone health and balanced hormones. Vitamin D3 has many roles in the human life is extensive (see bonus articles on my blog page www.fitnessforwardstudio.com/blog for more information on the role of Vitamin D. Even if we live in sunny climates, people often don't spend enough time outside in the natural light and fresh air.

Dr. Josh Axe and other practitioners suggest supplementing with *2,000 IU to 5,000 IU daily of Vitamin* D3 if not in the sun as vitamin deficiency is very common. Vitamin D is not a regular vitamin; it is a pro-hormone that you get from exposure to the sun or supplements.

- Vitamin D deficiency symptoms are a weakened immune system, gut infection as candida or bacterial overgrowth, emotional roller coaster, hormone imbalance, trouble putting on muscle or losing weight, weakened bones or teeth, cancer, heart disease, or diabetes.
- Vitamin D plays a role in the body to improve the immune response, digestive health, mood, bone health, hormone balance, and more.
- The causes of Vitamin D include not enough sunlight each day, toxic chemicals from BPA in plastic bottles.

- Make it your goal to get outside every day for about twenty to thirty minutes for natural sunlight while you are on your daily walk and the fresh air always offers additional benefits.
- Add foods with Vitamin D as wild caught fish, mushrooms, eggs, and raw fermented milk.
- Supplement with a high-quality D3 vitamin with fish oil or take a supplement with fat source as coconut oil, almond butter or avocado to aid in the absorption as Vitamin D is a fat-soluble vitamin. An essential supplement for most all of us. Even myself who trains in the outdoors most days of the week. Vitamin D is required for the hormone, immune system, emotional system, and bone health.

11. ***Get off birth control pills:*** the pill is a synthetic hormone that raises estrogen levels and linked too many health risks to increased risk of breast cancer, blood clotting, stroke, migraines, gallbladder disease, and more.

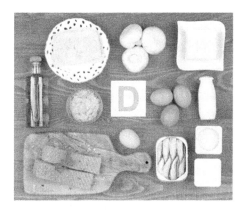

The big five WHOLESTIC Method Digestion tips for becoming a fat burner:

1. _____
2. _____
3. _____
4. _____
5. _____

The WHOLESTIC Method to improving fat loss, health and performance for life and sports by working from the inside out

Implement the tools you learn from this manual and my podcast episodes. The WHOLESTIC Method will provide you the tools to transform the WHOLE you by becoming a fat burner, optimizing your health, and improving performance for life and sports by working from the inside out.

RESOURCES:

http://tinyurl.com/WeightLossHoromones
www.bengreenfield.com
http://tinyurl.com/FatInfluencers
http://tinyurl.com/LeptinGherlin
http://tinyurl.com/HormonesMakeYouFat
www.chriskresser.com
http://www.amymyersmd.com

Learn More About Leaky Gut and Gut Repair:
http://tinyurl.com/DraxeLeakyGut
http://tinyurl.com/HealthfulElementsLeakyGut
http://tinyurl.com/KresserGutHealth
http://tinyurl.com/GapsDietInfo

Find more articles on:
http://tinyurl.com/HolickVitamanD
http://draxe.com/vitamin-d-deficiency/
http://draxe.com/vitamin-d-deficiency-symptoms/
http://tinyurl.com/VitaminDDeficiencies
http://tinyurl.com/VitaminDOsteo

To learn more about hormones and health:
http://draxe.com/4-steps-to-heal-leak
https://youtu.be/CVFA96t9G2I

http://wellnessmama.com/5425/balance-hormones/

http://draxe.com/10-ways-balance-hormones-naturally/

http://tinyurl.com/Top5BestFoods

https://www.youtube.com/watch?v=g-72k7h8WYI

ELEMENT #7
HYDRATION

We all know we need to be hydrated to stay healthy, but how does drinking more water improve our ability to burn fat and improve our performance? To be healthy from the inside out, we need to be adequately hydrated with natural clean water... not juice, coffee, soda, and other beverages. Remember that our body is around seventy-five percent (75%) water, and that while we can live for weeks without food, we can only survive for days without water. Water is essential for cellular homeostasis and for performing in daily life. The most important nutrient for our health may be water.

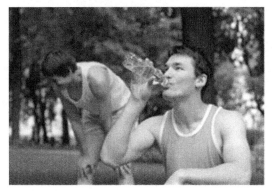

How much water do we need? It depends on climatic conditions, perspiration, medical conditions, exercise intensity and duration. You lose water through breath, perspiration, urine and bowel movements and for your body to function properly you must replenish its water supply. According to the Institute of Medicine, men should drink about 13 cups (3 liters) a day and women 9 cups (2.2 liters) a day. While most of us have heard the "Drink eight 8 ounce glasses a day" this is not supported by any evidence. That said, it is easy to remember and is an ok rule of thumb if you are in a temperate climate and not exercising intensely.

While getting enough water each day is critical to overall health, some people, mostly athletes, will over consume water and over hydrate. This can lead to a condition called hyponatremia, which is when the level of sodium in our blood is abnormally low. Sodium is an electrolyte and it helps regulate the amount of water in and around your cells. Because you lose sodium through sweat, Hyponatremia can result from drinking too much water during endurance sports/races which dilutes the sodium content of the blood. Drinking too much water at other times can also cause low sodium. According to the Mayo Clinic, when sodium levels are diluted, this can cause the water levels to rise and the cells to swell which can cause mild to life-threatening health problems.

Dr. Tim Noakes is the author of *Waterlogged* (and *The Real Meal Revolution* and we did a podcast on see www.thewholeathletepodcast.com archives) and has done abundant research on over-hydration, electrolytes, hyponatremia, and health. So be sure to check him this out for more information.

THE WATER CURE

Another book, *Your Body's Many Cries for Water,* by F. Batmanghelidj, M.D., is an easy read everyone should review if they have any type of health issues. His research shows that Unintentional Chronic Dehydration (UCD) contributes to and even produces pain and many degenerative diseases that could be prevented with proper hydration.

What he has found is a simple solution to many of our health problems - drink more water to hydrate the body. We don't treat thirst with medications and we shouldn't treat dehydration related aches and pains with pills either. Now Big Pharma would much prefer you take a pill and fulfills the "I don't want to change anything to get better" paradigm of our culture. As we have said throughout this book, rather than treat symptoms, it is far better to search for the root cause of the problem according to Dr. Batmanghelidj could be dehydration.

The quote at the beginning of the book is the perfect fit:

"The significant problems we have cannot be solved at the same level of thinking with which we created them."
- Albert Einstein

Dr. Batmanghelidj says, "You are not sick; you are thirsty. Don't treat thirst with medications." Most of his recommendations are based on personal experience and research, but as I've said, it wouldn't hurt us all to drink more water each day. I drink water throughout the day, but even I need to drink more than I do and that doesn't happen unless I carry my water bottle with me in the car, at work, during workouts, and at meals. So, I highly recommend you get a reusable water bottle to keep with you as a reminder to drink water. Oh, and for the health of the planet, avoid buying bottled water and this means in the airport, as well. Take your bottle with you and fill it from the water fountain once you are past security.

I also suggest reading *Your Body's Many Cries for Water* to learn about how dehydration impacts your performance in life and sports. Staying hydrated may not solve or cure every health problem, but we should try to improve symptoms by drinking more *clean* water as most people are chronically dehydrated and don't know it.

HYDRATION AND THE BODY

Among other things, staying properly hydrated helps in lubricating the joints, maintaining normal electrical properties of cells, and removing toxic waste. The colon, brain, heart and in fact every cell of our body needs proper hydration to function correctly. And don't get me started on digestion. So much constipation could be resolved with proper hydration. Instead, people eat more fiber without the proper amount of water, making matters worse. Either that or they take a laxative which can provide temporary relief at the expense of further dehydration. Obviously, water and hydration play many important roles in our blood, lymph nodes, digestive juices, urine, tears, and sweat.

According to the Nutritional Therapy Association, some specific roles of water include:

- Improves oxygen delivery to cells
- Transports nutrients
- Enables cellular hydration
- Moistens oxygen for easier breathing
- Cushions bones and joints
- Absorbs shocks to joints and organs
- Regulates body temperature
- Removes wastes
- Flushes toxins
- Prevents tissues from sticking
- Lubricates joints
- Improves cell-to-cell communications

Unfortunately, dehydration is a major issue for many people. However, few people know that water loss of two percent (2%) of body weight can cause fatigue and a decrease of ten percent (10%) of body weight can cause health problems including digestion, immune, cardiovascular, and musculoskeletal. Even more frightening is a loss of more than ten percent (10%) may cause death. A friend's cousin died from dehydration while hiking one hot summer day in Arizona. It is a fact.

Another fact is our body can only produce eight percent (8%) of its daily requirements via metabolic processes so we must get the remaining ninety-two percent (92%) of our water needs via the food and beverages we consume each day. So, keep your bottle on your desk, in your car, and near you during workouts, especially when you are outdoors in hot weather or at high altitudes.

ALL WATER ARE NOT EQUAL

Which beverages or types of water keep us hydrated? Should we drink mineral water, distilled water, tap water, filtered water? For example, I love sparkling water and filtered water and have purchased distilled water as well.

Most of our tap water is contaminated with bacteria, chlorine, fluoride, bacteria, parasites, pesticides, solvents, and heavy metals. Municipal drinking water is often contaminated with agricultural chemicals and over 700 pollutants, according to the EPA. The biggest polluter of our water (rivers and streams), as reported by the EPA, is the commercial agriculture farmers. Dr. Mercola notes that glyphosate, the active ingredient in Roundup, has been detected in the groundwater in Spain. And this was in 2012. A report released by As You Sow states that glyphosate is ubiquitous in the environment as they are used on America's largest crops including corn, soy, canola, sugar beets, and cotton, and sprayed on wheat as a pre-harvest agent. In addition, prescribed medications have found their way into our water supply via excrement, urine and a flush of the toilet. An EPA study tested for 56 drugs including oxycodone, blood pressure meds and common over the counter drugs such as Tylenol and ibuprofen. More than half the samples tested positive for at least twenty-five of the drugs monitored.

"We were surprised to find that many drugs occurring across all the wastewater plants," said Mitchell Kostich, the EPA research biologist who led the study. "We were also surprised to see so many drugs of a particular class—the high blood pressure medications—appear at those levels across the board."

Given that news, I believe everyone should test their own tap water for bacteria count, mineral content, and amount of chemical pollutants. Ideally, we would all install a filtration or another type of purification system in our houses or find another source of drinking water other than from the tap. Our skin is a mouth, so be aware of contaminated water in your shower.

Distilled water come from the process of turning water into steam and removing most minerals, organisms, and chemicals from the water. Thus distilled water has no minerals and because of this has the special property of being able to actively absorb toxins from the body and eliminate them. Studies validate the benefits of drinking distilled water during a short cleanse or detox. Also, a good time to drink distilled water is when you are heating it up for herbal teas as the medicinal properties of the water will be pulled out more than regular water.

On the flip side, distilled water may attract other minerals in the body so it would not be ideal for someone who may already be slightly deficient in minerals as it may cause more mineral deficiency. Fasting using distilled water can be dangerous because of the rapid loss of electrolytes (sodium, potassium, chloride) and trace minerals like magnesium, deficiencies of which can cause heart palpations and high blood pressure. Cooking foods in distilled water pulls the minerals out of them and lowers their nutrient value. Drinking distilled water absorbs carbon dioxide, making it acidic and not ideal for drinking.

Ideally, I would like to see *Reverse Osmosis* (RO) filtration systems with remineralization cartridges in our homes, schools, and workplaces to protect us from contaminated water. Note: while RO systems do a great job filtering, they also remove the minerals and without the remineralizing, they have the same adverse effects as distilled water.

Dr. Mercola recommends a whole house water filter that has three separate stages of contamination removal:

- Stage one removes sediment.
- Stage two removes chlorine and heavy metals.
- Stage three should be a heavy-duty carbon filter for removing hormones, drug residues, chemicals, pesticides, and herbicides.

You want to look for granular carbon in the carbon filter, not a solid block of carbon. The granular carbon allows for better water flow, which translates to more water pressure and better filtering properties as well.

WATER ADDITIVES AND ALTERNATIVES

A study carried out at the University of Aberdeen Medical School found that some fruit and vegetables may hydrate the body twice as effectively as a glass of water. Water-rich fruit and vegetables provide mineral salts, natural sugars, amino acids and vitamins that are lost in exercise and help hydrate people more effectively than water or sports drinks. A University of Naples study found plant chemicals (lutein and zeaxanthin) found in watermelon and papaya help boost hydration even further. Due to the water and mineral balance, a cucumber can produce similar hydration levels to twice the volume of water while providing ideal levels of calcium, magnesium, potassium, sodium and other minerals. Celery is another hydration star.

A much more popular way of getting the benefits of hydrating fruits and vegetables is to add them to a pitcher of water. Cucumber water is particularly popular and is a thirst-quenching, hydrating, vitamin and mineral powerhouse. In addition, cucumbers contain an anti-inflammatory flavonol called *Fisetin*. As we know from all of our discussions here, the anti-inflammatory is good.

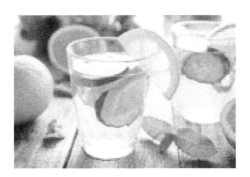

Another option is to add a sprinkle of good source sea salt in your morning water. This provides essential minerals to help retain the water and this is really useful when you are outside in hot climates. The salt, whether in our water or food, helps the cells retain the water and is especially important if you are suffering from adrenal fatigue or taking diuretics. Sodium regulates the amount of water held outside the cells so salt isn't always a bad word. Also, remember that dehydration is also a source of stress to the body—or rather the brain—so make sure you don't add another stressor to your body. Stay hydrated as it is an easy solution to many of our health and body complaints.

A little-known gem is called Crystal Energy, created by the genius inventor Dr. Patrick Flanagan. It is a form of colloidal silica found in glacial waters around the world and when added to your water it instantly structures water into a highly organized liquid crystal. This arrangement more closely matches how water surrounds the cells in the body. Dr. Flanagan's studies have shown that Crystal Energy lowers water molecules' surface tension thereby helping to increase the flow across cell membranes. With the increased rate of water flow, cellular hydration, nutrient transport, and toxin elimination are increased. In addition, it makes the water taste delicious

ATHLETES AND THE LIQUID CONSUMPTION MYTH

We used to tell athletes to drink often during workouts, before you are thirsty, to improve performance and achieve optimal health. Now it is said that we need to drink when we are thirsty. I used to force myself to drink a bottle of water per hour and consume 300-500 calories per hour during my Ironman races when I started racing in 2001. All it did was make my belly bloated which forced me to eliminate these excess fluids while I continued to race (also known as throwing up to feel better). I used to set a timer to drink every fifteen minutes during an Ironman race or marathon just because I thought I was supposed to.

Who told us to drink and eat that much per hour? It was likely the sports drink and food industry companies. Don't get me started as this problem is similar to the entire food pyramid, cholesterol/heart disease, diabetes guidelines, and heart association guidelines. Just look who is funding these organizations that are supposed to be helping to cure disease. Actually, they work on how to keep you alive longer, not on how to prevent or reverse disease. They recommend the very foods and beverages that have been clinically shown to cause cancer, diabetes and heart disease. There is a similar graphic for big pharma contributions. Don't trust them.

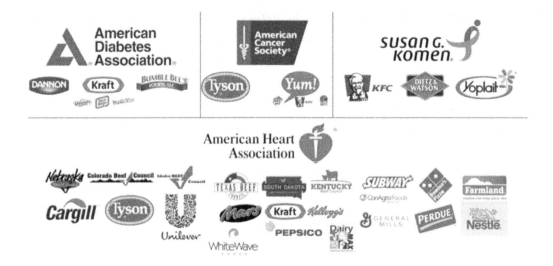

So who can we trust to get the correct guidelines to help us reach our optimal health levels and peak performance for life and sports? Go to the Dark Side and listen to the underground news without the influence of big companies funding the research to create guidelines. I recommend spending a little time and vetting your source though as even these folks can be quacks. Gaia.com is a "Netflix for Awakening People" and has tons of evidence-based information on health and government corruption.

ELECTROLYTES

Electrolytes are minerals in our body that produce an electrically conducting solution when dissolved in water. For example, table salt (Sodium Chloride) dissolved in water dissociates into its component positive ion of sodium (Na+) and negative ion of chloride (Cl-). Our heart, muscle and nerve cells use electrolytes to maintain voltages across their cell membranes and to carry electrical impulses to other cells. This process relies on the balance of this electrically charged fluid between the inside and outside of our cells. We need to have just the right amount of electrolytes as they regulate our nerve and muscle function, hydration, blood pH, blood pressure, as well as rebuilding damaged tissue. To maintain constant electrolyte concentrations in our body fluids, electrolytes must be replaced by eating fresh fruits and vegetables and consuming sea salt. Any excess electrolytes are filtered out by our kidneys. The optimal amount of electrolyte levels varies per person and depends on changes due to sweating, kidney problems, medication, vomiting or diarrhea.

There are seven major electrolytes essential to life:

- Sodium (Na+)
- Chloride (Cl-)
- Potassium (K+)
- Magnesium (Mg++)
- Calcium (Ca++)
- Phosphate (HPO4-)
- Bicarbonate (HCO3-)

Each electrolyte has a critical role in keeping our cells and body functioning at optimal levels when in the right balance. Again, as I say for almost every topic and in my book, MORE IS NOT BETTER in most situations. As with our entire body systems, we are on a teeter-totter, balancing to stay in equilibrium. Too much of anything can be toxic while too little can lead to deficiencies.

SODIUM

Let's dive into the role of sodium. Sodium helps control the amount of water in and around our cells, regulating blood volume, maintaining muscle, and assisting nerve function. Sodium is the major positively charged ion outside your cells and is mostly found in blood, plasma and lymph fluid and creates part of our electrical pump to keep electrolytes in balance inside and outside our cells. Too much sodium leads to what is called hypernatremia (also known as dehydration) and too little leads to hyponatremia.

Most sodium comes from consuming table salt and we need at least 500 mg per day with a recommended intake of around two grams. Please use quality Sea salt or Himalayan salt, both of which contain trace minerals such as calcium, iron, and magnesium that are essential for proper body function. The processed table salts have been bleached and stripped of their natural minerals, and may contain toxic stabilizers.

CHLORIDE

Chloride is the major negative ion and is primarily found in the extracellular fluid. It works closely with sodium to maintain proper balance and pressure of the various fluid compartments in the body. Chloride is vital for maintaining proper pH in the body and is also obtained through salt intake.

POTASSIUM

While sodium is found mostly outside cells, potassium is the major ion inside cells and is critical for regulating heartbeat and muscle function. It forms the other half of the electrical pump keeping electrolytes in balance. We take in potassium by eating fruits and vegetables, grass-fed meats, and organic poultry. Coconut water is another great source of potassium. The balance of sodium and potassium is important, and an imbalance can increase the risk of hypertension and heart disease.

MAGNESIUM

It is estimated that more than seventy-five percent (75%) of Americans are deficient in magnesium. This under-appreciated substance is necessary for over 300 biochemical reactions in the body and plays an important role in the synthesis of DNA and RNA. It helps maintain normal nerve and muscle function, boosts the immune system, and stabilizes stable heart rate and blood sugar. Nuts and leafy green vegetables are a good source of magnesium as is coffee and tea. Rubbing magnesium oil over your kidneys before bed can assist in your magnesium intake and help you sleep while taking magnesium malate supplements will bond any aluminum in your body (the malic acid binds with the aluminum and is excreted).

CALCIUM

Calcium is needed for the formation of bones and teeth, as well as transmission of nerve impulses, blood clotting, and muscle contraction. It is the most abundant mineral in your body and deficiency can lead to osteoporosis. Fortunately, the list of calcium-rich foods is long and varied. Yes, you get from dairy though also from dark leafy greens, bok choy, non-GMO soy, okra, broccoli, green beans, almonds, and sardines, to name a few.

PHOSPHATE

Phosphate is the second most abundant mineral in your body and eighty-five percent (85%) of it is found in your bones. It works closely with calcium to strengthen bones and teeth and is also essential to energy production in the cells, tissue growth, and repair and is a building block for DNA and cell membranes. While most people get enough in their diet, pumpkin and squash seeds, salmon, nuts, and shellfish are examples of foods with phosphate.

BICARBONATE

Bicarbonate is part of the pH balancing system. When acids build up through the metabolic processes or production of lactic acid in your muscles, the kidneys release bicarbonate to counteract the acidity. It is secreted by the stomach during digestion and when ingested, for example, with mineral water, helps buffer lactic acid and other acidic conditions in the body.

STAYING HYDRATED

If you are like most people, you wake up and drink coffee until lunch, then you drink soda, and later, you have wine or a cocktail at dinner time. We think we are drinking water throughout the day, but most of my coaching clients end up drinking a few glasses a day which is not the recommended amount as I've stated before.

While one size does not fit all, the best way to ensure that you are staying hydrated is to keep 32-ounce bottle of water on your desk and commit to drinking at least two of these. This will satisfy the 8 x 8 ounces though as we have seen more is recommended. Note that room temperature water is recommended. If you drink cold water, you may feel it jiggle in your tummy while sits in your belly warming to room temperature. Another option is to get a water tracking app on your smartphone or tablet. These apps can be programmed to remind you to drink and can be used to track your intake. And remember, the other items you drink, like iced tea, coffee, juices, or other high sugar beverages don't count as your water intake. Keep in mind that we lose water throughout the day simply by breathing. Even if you are not exercising that day, you still need to drink your water and stay hydrated.

I always tell my personal training and coaching clients that we must build a strong stable foundation before we can build the house. We can all start drinking more water throughout the day (filtered clean water) as part of the quest to own our health and by taking a preventative approach to our personal health care. By staying hydrated you may even feel better from ailments such as arthritis, headaches, digestion, and even depression.

If you want to continue your journey to becoming a WHOLESTIC athlete to improve fat loss, health, and performance, we need to look outside the box, avoid the new fads from mainstream media, and research the facts. We need to take our health into our hands and make it our responsibility to become healthy from the inside out.

The big five WHOLESTIC Method Hydration tips for becoming a fat burner:

1. _____
2. _____
3. _____
4. _____
5. _____

The WHOLESTIC Method to improving fat loss, health and performance for life and sports by working from the inside out.

REFERENCES:

http://tinyurl.com/WaterHydrationHealth
http://tinyurl.com/HydrationWaterFacts
http://tinyurl.com/FluidElectrolyte
www.medicalnewstoday.com/articles
http://tinyurl.com/ImportanceHydration
http://tinyurl.com/CompetingInHeat

1. Electrolytes, Potassium, Sodium, Chloride, and Bicarbonate Information. What Are Electrolytes? Fit Health & Discovery (2012). http://tinyurl.com/ElectrolytesRef2
2. Sodium (Na) in Blood. WebMD (2010). http://tinyurl.com/ElectrolytesRef3
3. Johnson, Larry E. Electrolytes: Electrolyte Balance: Merck Manual Home Edition (2008). http://tinyurl.com/ElectrolytesRef4
4. Armstrong, Larry. Magnesium Deficiency & Alcohol. Livestrong.com (2010). http://tinyurl.com/ElectrolytesRef5
5. Electrolyte Balance. Nano-Cal (2005). http://tinyurl.com/ElectrolytesRef6

ELEMENT #8
HAPPINESS

Probably the most important element of The WHOLESTIC Method is *happiness*. As with all the eight elements, if one is off balance, the rest of the elements are thrown out of alignment. If we are truly happy, we eat better, exercise more, sleep better, lower our stress, etc. At the other end of the spectrum, if we eat too much sugar and gluten/grains that cause distress in our bodies and brains, then we are not happy campers. If we are stressed out at work, home, and our life duties, we are usually not happy. If we are not sleeping well, we are unhappy and/or grumpy.

Did you know that feeling happy is connected to burning fat? Well, it is and we are going to find out how in this chapter. Subjective (self-assessed) well-being is not well understood though it may affect our health through behaviors as well as through immune and cardiovascular systems. Happy people tend to move and exercise more and also tend to have healthier lifestyles in general.

How many people do you know that battle depression? I continue to hear about more people who are depressed and on anti-depressants. It turns out what we eat makes a difference to our mood and leaky gut, digestion issues, and inflammation can drastically influence how you feel both physically and emotionally.

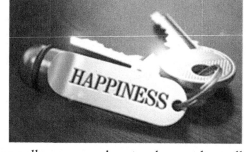

If you are addicted to sugar, as many people are in our society, you may find yourself with major mood swings as your blood sugar levels spike high then crash low. As Vinnie Tortorich says, you can eliminate the blood sugar roller coaster by simply avoiding all processed sugars and grains.

Now, how does our happiness impact or influence our health and the other elements in The WHOLESTIC Method? My goal is to help everyone realize we need to improve the WHOLE person from the inside out to be healthy, not just to exercise more, move more, and eat less. If it was that easy, we wouldn't have so many unhealthy, overweight, unhappy individuals in our country and the world.

From my experience, we can't improve fat loss, health, and performance with only one element. Happiness is just as important in improving health and is part of managing our stress and sleeping better. In this chapter, we will look at becoming more focused and in the moment. I believe in the need to disconnect and unplug. Do you depend on happiness by checking out social media posts and feeds? Perhaps our constant glorification to be busy, need to multi-task, and our addiction to the fear of missing out on social media (FOMA) is influencing our level of happiness.

I do believe that if we are chronically stressed, anxious, and tired, we are going to be less happy about our life which may impact our food choices, exercise, sleep, digestion, movement, and more. I created The WHOLESTIC Method with the eight elements that are all interconnected; one element impacts the other and if one is off then the domino effect occurs. To be a healthy happy individual from the inside out, we must start working on the WHOLE person internally instead of the external superficial layer. We need to take the time to go inward and discover what makes us happy, moves our soul and drives us to be excited to wake up another day.

HAPPINESS DEFINED

Happiness is a mental or emotional state of well-being defined by positive or pleasant emotions ranging from contentment to intense joy. [1] Happy mental states may also reflect judgments by a person about their overall well-being. [2] A variety of biological, psychological, economic, religious, and philosophical approaches have striven to define happiness and identify its sources. Various research groups, including positive psychology and happiness economics, are employing the scientific method to research questions about what happiness is, and how it might be attained.

The United Nations declared 20 March the International Day of Happiness to recognize the relevance of happiness and well-being as universal goals.

In reality, happiness is a subjective state. What makes one person happy may make another miserable. Some people love skiing, others are miserable in the cold. Still, others love lying on the beach and others find it boring. I would argue that true happiness consists of a life of consistent enthusiasm, joy, gratitude, and contentment. Temporary elation or infatuation, followed by ho-hum is not necessarily a happy life. People often think they are happy when they find a new love when in reality this state is hormone and ego driven and eventually wears off. I would say most people look for something outside of themselves to "make" them happy when in reality happiness is something that cannot be found outside and always starts on the inside. A happy inside attracts happy outer circumstances.

FINDING HAPPINESS

Do you wake up happy or grumpy? Do you have mood swings throughout the day? I notice at least one person each day walk into my studio door with a frown on their face, upset about the traffic or a negative experience. Is our life really that bad that we need to get worked up about a situation or person? As my husband says, those are first world problems. Is it because they didn't sleep well, didn't eat the right foods (sugar and gluten.), and/or they are too stressed from demands of daily life? Probably all the above.

According to the author and speaker, Eckhart Tolle, many people who choose to seek the spiritual path do so because they are unhappy or desperately miserable. They have lived a life that lacks meaning, feels empty and is filled with anger or anguish. He points out that whether mild or severe, pain itself is a great motivator when it comes to choosing to grow psychologically and spiritually. He offers a few steps to becoming happier.

Understand why we are unhappy. We are usually unhappy because we are trapped in the small, limited confines of our ego and identified with a false self that is not who we really are. The ego is endlessly preoccupied with past and future, the past causing worry and the future anxiety. Understanding this will help to liberate you from your ego and its trappings.

Accept what is. The great Indian philosopher and spiritual teacher J. Krishnamurti expressed this secret in a lecture he gave near the end of his life. He said to his audience, "Do you want to know my secret? ... My secret is that I don't mind what happens." So, try saying to yourself "I don't mind what happens" or "Whatever is happing in this moment is okay."

Letting go of judgment. When we accept and align with what is, we are not resigning ourselves to a fate we may or may not like and that we largely have no control over. We are empowering ourselves with peace and a sense of clarity that will allow us to make non-reactive choices about our present conditions.

In general, we want to observe our ego and the voice inside of our head, judging, comparing, resisting what is going on and then complaining. We want to respond rather than react. Pay attention to body sensations. To you feel them in your solar plexus, heart or throat? Is the emotion anger, sadness, frustration? Going inside to notice your state will take you a long way toward a happier you. I highly recommend reading *The Power of Now* and *The New Earth* by Eckhart Tolle. These are amazing reads and will help you recognize the happiness blocking ego that all humans have.

HAPPINESS THROUGH FOOD

Anna Vocino is a comic voice-over actor, podcaster, and now a cookbook author of *Eat Happy*. Anna points out that people eat because they want to make themselves happy. When questioned about what brought her to write a cookbook, she revealed that when she was twenty-eight, she was diagnosed with celiac disease and she had to give up gluten to ease her pain. After that, she decided to convert her favorite recipes into gluten, sugar and grain-free versions so that she could continue to enjoy her meals. In her cookbook, Anna introduces delicious sugar-free food with the intent to help people realize that processed food is not good for health or happiness. Too often people buy convenient processed food from the grocery store that is easy and quick to prepare if any preparation is required at all. The thing is, there are recipes that can be prepared at home in less than an hour or even half an hour that is healthy and satisfying. Anna created the cookbook to make people happy with the amazing food that supports the NSNG (No Sugar No Grains) way of living that Vinnie Tortorich and Anna discuss on their podcast. For years, Anna and Vinnie have discussed the importance of NSNG; avoid sugar and grains if you want to feel good, look good, and be happy from the inside and out.

People who travel a lot spend often eat in restaurants and hotels though when they get home they do not bother to cook food and continue to eat out. There is a huge quality difference between restaurant food and the food cooked at home. Anna's cookbook is filled with food for every type of eater and satisfies a variety of cravings that make them a happy camper... everyone can find dozens of delicious recipes in her *Eat Happy* cookbook.

Anna's experience with having celiac disease motivated her to write the cookbook, but it is also based on what sugar and grains do to people's mood, gut, and entire body. Honestly, most people are not aware of or know how messed up they are from eating sugar and grains. Anna used to have horrible seasonal allergies and when she took gluten, sugar, and grains out of her diet, her allergies eventually cleared up. She was relieved to have gotten rid of her health problems by changing to her NSNG eating plan, lifestyle, and avoiding any medication.

Anna teaches people to cook food at home and have fun doing it. She stresses inviting friends and family over for happy gatherings. Anna thought most restaurants use low-quality oil and kept cooking food all day in the same grease without bothering to change it.

What made Anna call her cookbook *Eat Happy*? She thought by creating recipes and meal that are without sugar and grains, her meals would make people's life easier with less stress (simple and easy to make recipes for even people as myself who can't cook.) and happier (less sugar = less mood swings). Cooking with Anna's recommended recipes will bring happiness and joy to people's life mostly because they are no longer on the blood sugar roller coaster and they are avoiding foods that make them feel crappy and unhappy.

Happiness is a choice we have in life. No one else can make you happy unless you decide to make yourself happy. If you want to be happy and live a beautiful life, start by changing your food plan today. Try avoiding sugar and grains (gluten). Choose what is good for your body, nourishment for the soul. Good, clean food will make you happy.

HAPPINESS, SMILING, AND LOVING OURSELVES

Do you say hello or smile when you pass someone, even when no one else is around? Since Christmas/New Year's family vacation in Florida in 1999, I noticed how everyone greeted each other on my morning runs. Why was everyone happy and smiling? I realized when a total stranger said hello to me when we passed each other on the boardwalk, *I felt happy*. Now, I always make sure I wave or say good morning or good afternoon on my workouts. When I do any type of race or event, I make sure I cheer on the other participants when we pass each other and always thank the volunteers for their hard work. When I smile, have fun, laugh, I am more relaxed and happy. The happier I am, the more the people around me will be, as well, and they'll feel more at ease, relaxed, and happy, too.

It turns out there is a physiological reason we feel good when we smile or are smiled at. Smiling activates the release of neuropeptides that help reduces stress and facilitate messaging to the whole body. And since smiling causes the release of dopamine, endorphins, and serotonin, our whole body can feel, great. These endorphins also act as a natural pain reliever and anti-depressant. The interesting part is that being smiled at activates the same areas of the brain, so smiling at someone is a win-win for all parities.

Many years ago, when I worked in fitness management at a private athletic club in a hotel (The Bellevue Club), I always remembered the 10 & 5 Hospitality Rule and I continue to practice this rule in my own daily life. I think we should all practice this and pay it forward by acknowledging total strangers when you pass by them:

ZONE OF HOSPITALITY: THE 10 & 5 RULE:

- Anytime a guest is within ten feet of a staff member, the staff member should make eye contact with a warm smile to acknowledge the oncoming guests.

- When a staff member is approximately five feet from a guest, a sincere greeting or friendly gesture of acknowledgment should accompany the eye contact and smile.
- At Walt Disney World, Disney cast members nearing a guest must follow Disney's Seven Service Guidelines:
  1. Make eye contact and smile
  2. Greet and welcome each and every guest
  3. Seek out guest contact
  4. Provide immediate service recovery
  5. Display appropriate body language at all times
  6. Preserve the magical guest experience
  7. Thank each and every guest

Is it any wonder why we are all smiling, laughing, and happy at the Magic Kingdom? When I was there I had the happy grinning face of a five-year-old walking even though it was hot and crowded. My childhood memories I cherished of our summer vacations at Disneyland made me smile and happy. Why is Disneyland the happiest place on Earth? Maybe it's as simple as the customer service and the way they treat their guests.

I remember my seventh-grade math teacher had a poster in his classroom that was in our face every day:

Bring a PMA = Positive Mental Attitude

Maybe because it was math class, which was not always a favorite school subject for most of us, though I am sure the teacher was on to something. As a youth, we play, smile, laugh, and cry and were open with our emotions. What happened as we grew up and got older? Did we get too serious and become too negative? Had my math teacher already figured out that we, as a society, needed to improve our attitude toward life each day? Why do many of us become uptight, stressed, and anxious as we grow up instead of being silly, laughing, and enjoying every day in the moment?

A longtime client and friend wrote what happiness means to being healthy:

Each of us has goals and dreams of finding happiness and good health. In an ever-changing world, with the constant demand we place on ourselves to achieve in both our personal relationships and our contributions in our work, often we put off what is needed for ourselves to live a happier and healthier life. Setting realistic goals and breaking negative patterns in our lives is paramount to the success of this journey. It requires not only looking outward to measure our progress, but also to look deeply inward to understanding who we are.

Though more complex, it is far more rewarding to find acceptance of yourself as a person. Understanding and appreciating who you are and changing the negative patterns of behavior that follow us will result in improved overall health. But, more importantly, it will create a brighter emotional outcome that can sustain you throughout your life. Being really good to myself, family, friends, and community have led me to a path of self-acceptance. I feel good about my prospects moving ahead. Eating well and exercising to stay fit has become much easier over time. I've discovered real progress in many aspects of my life.

~ Josh Beloff, husband, and father of two

I wrote a blog a few years back entitled *Are You Living Life or Just Living?* I have become more aware of people's lack of happiness each day, as well as negative self-talk and programming. Self-talk is often skewed toward the negative and often it is just plain wrong and based on false beliefs that we acquired through childhood trauma. It is important to spend some time understanding these false beliefs by first recognizing that they exist and are indeed not true, then trying to understand where they came from. There is a great book by Bryan Hubbard called "The Untrue Story of You: how to Let Go of the Past" that may help you find your way around these false beliefs. Bryan presents a powerful, groundbreaking theory explaining who we really are, how our relationship to our past affects us and how we can finally find true healing and happiness. Finally, we can reprogram these false beliefs into more true statements such as "I count, I matter in this life," "I am loved and I am loveable." The list goes on. Mirror work (looking in the mirror and telling yourself that you are valuable and loved) can be difficult in the beginning though through time will become easier. You may not even notice that your life has become easier and happier as you love yourself fully. This simple (though not necessarily easy) technique can be learned from the late master or mirror work Louise Hay in her book, *Mirror Work: 21 Days to Heal Your Life.*

Earlier in this manual, I talked about the SweetBeat HRV stress monitor iPhone app to monitor your stress, exercise recovery, and daily heart rate variability. Doing an HRV session is a great opportunity to relax, unplug, and breathe. Taking time out for yourself provides space for finding happiness within. As I always say, you can't love other people until you love yourself. If you are not happy with who you are, then how can you truly love another and live each day to the fullest?

I found an interesting article online Harvard School of Public Health website on *The biology of emotion—and what it may teach us about helping people to live longer.* Could a sunny outlook mean fewer colds and less heart disease? The experts say yes.

KEYS TO A HAPPIER LIFE

Being present in each moment is difficult at best and has been accomplished only by a few masters throughout history. That said, we need to do daily work on our mindset in order to focus and be present. The voice in our head, mostly fueled by the selfish righteous ego is generally in charge, always in the past or future and never in the present. The thing is, the present is all there is. The past is made up of an accumulation of present moments and the future does not exist yet and is malleable and uncertain. Still, our mind is rarely right here right now and this is true for all but a few rare humans. As mentioned previously, the past causes worry and the future anxiety. Being present in the moment and, importantly, not resisting what is happening in the moment will take you a long way through your evolution and journey of experiencing happiness. Remember to read Eckhart Tolle's books if you want to grow in presence and learn to spot and ignore the cunning ego.

Many of you may be familiar with the hit movie and book The Secret. While the movie is designed to reach the typical "consumer" mindset, it is a gem and introduces some very important truths. Everything in the Universe is vibrating. Everything. Your thoughts and emotions have a frequency as well (you can see them on a brain scan called an EEG). Different emotions have a different frequency and once you learn some presence you can then *choose* how you are going to *respond* to a given situation and thus choose the frequency that you will be emitting. Gratitude is one of the easiest ways to start to shift your vibration. Those of us reading this book are in the privileged few on the planet and have plenty to be grateful for. Getting in the habit of giving thanks for what you have will lead to habitual gratitude and a gradual change in your circumstances and happiness. You will smile more and create an atmosphere of joy that your family and friends will also get to experience. I highly recommend The Secret book which is less sensationalized than the movie though I do recommend the movie as well.

I saved a giveaway bag from a race because I love the sayings printed on it. It has positive living quotes similar to what Lululemon started with their packaging and marketing:

- Mindset attitude
- Stay positive and grab the bull by the horns
- Find your voice
- Own your tomorrow
- Giving back to the community creates change
- We are all one people
- Slow down and unplug
- Find what makes you happy. If you love what you do, work isn't work

- There will always be ups and downs; don't lose your direction
- Equally as important to invest in people
- Take ownership of the Human Experience; find your passion and get involved
- Be a lifelong learner; find something that wakes you up.
- Travel journeys and experience living history
- Find the experience that inspires you

Research suggests that certain personal attributes—whether inborn or shaped by positive life circumstances—help some people avoid or healthfully manage diseases such as heart attacks, strokes, diabetes, and depression.

These include:

- Emotional vitality: a sense of enthusiasm, hopefulness, engagement
- Optimism: the perspective that good things will happen, and that one's actions account for the good things that occur in life
- Supportive networks of family and friends
- Being good at **self-regulation**, i.e. bouncing back from stressful challenges and knowing that things will eventually look up again; choosing healthy behaviors such as physical activity and eating well; and avoiding risky behaviors such as unsafe sex, drinking alcohol to excess, and regular overeating.

I love the concept self-regulation as well as making more wellness deposits in order to be happy. If you are happy, then people will want to be around you as you make them smile and laugh. A happy smile and laughter are contagious. I have been working on lowering my stress levels by taking more time each day to push pause and reset or do what I sometimes call recalibrate. While this sounds simple, it is not easy. It requires self-awareness and presence. If you don't notice that you have become slightly impatient, agitated, judgmental or stressed then you wouldn't know that a pause or reset is in order. I suggest setting an hourly timer to move, breathe and self-assess.

Once you have developed awareness of your inner state, you can determine how to self-regulate in an ongoing fashion which, I can guarantee, will lead to more happiness, calm and joy. I discovered that I felt guilty if I wasn't constantly doing something and after much self-reflection realize that it is okay for me to take care of myself. If I need to, I go home to my sanctuary and work at my home office instead of being visible at my studio. I take care of myself by going for my bike ride or run in the afternoon. This makes me a happier person for my evening clients and allows for an enjoyable atmosphere for all. I get a good night sleep so that my morning clients will have a good experience. Who wants to train with a grumpy and irritable coach who did not get enough sleep? Nobody I know.

Here is a story from one of my fellow teammates Todd Durkin Mastermind:

One of my daily morning rituals is to listen to my Daily Devotional with Rick Warren over at Saddleback Church. One of the episodes, he made a point that really stuck out to me which I'll explain it as soon as I tell this story…

I was at an ATM at Chase Bank last Friday and the guy in front of me was trying to withdraw some funds. After three attempts, he still couldn't do it and I was getting a bit antsy as I was short on time. As I peeked over to see what was going on, it repeatedly told him he had <u>insufficient funds</u>. He kept trying over and over again and the result was the same. And, this is what I remembered after listening to one of Rick's podcast and the big lesson: **You Can't Withdraw What You Haven't Deposited.**

You cannot take out more than you put in. This goes for every area of life and you will see it show up everywhere. People want to get extraordinary results within weeks or a couple of months. What they are really trying to do is withdraw more than they deposited. I have experienced this many times before when I would start something and work hard for a bit and expect there to be amazing results. Time and failures taught me I will only be able to take out what I put in and building extraordinary things take a lot of putting in toward that account (body, business, relationships, yourself,).

The work you do today will show in the future, but you can only do it **today**. You can't do tomorrow's work today.

Ask yourself:
- Where in your life do you want to withdraw more than you deposited?
- Where can you deposit more so you can get what you want in the future?
- Are you expecting to make a small deposit and take a big withdrawal in your health and fitness?
- Rather than looking at days or weeks, ask yourself what you're committed to depositing in the next year.
- Write the script of your life and recognize that it will take deposits to get the withdrawals you want.
- I have a poster on my wall and it says: **Design The Life You Deserve Because You Deserve the Life You Designed**

Happiness comes to different people in different ways. Some need to spend more quality time with friends and family each week as well as quality time with their spouse or partner. Others may actually find relief from unplugging each day for a few hours and even for a full day each week. I have become more aware of our society's obsession electronic devices and being continuously and overly connected. I encourage you to start observing how people behave when standing in line, when eating meals, driving their car or even while working out. Many are increasingly abusing the use of their phones, computers, and social media, so much that they have forgotten how to be present with each other and focus on conversations. I challenge you to make some changes to find happiness within yourself including:

- Unplugging each night when you get home from your day or at least one to two hours before bed
- Take one weekend day to stay off-line = no computer, cell phone or electronic devices
- Pick up the phone and call your friend instead of text them
- Schedule time with friends once a month or more that make you laugh and smile
- Take five minutes each day to meditate your own way if it is testing your HRV on our app, going for a nature walk without your phone or music or humming in your car while you drive somewhere that makes you happy.
- Schedule a day to yourself to be by yourself... a spa day, a walk or even a retreat out of town.

Happiness starts from inside you. Take time out to determine what daily practices bring you joy and happiness. How can you eliminate or change the negativity you may have in your life? Start by reprogramming what you say to yourself as well as aloud to your peers and become aware of what you feel on the inside. It may be time to take the armor down and share your emotions. Quoting the airline analogy, you may need to start putting the oxygen mask on your face before you start helping others. I found this quote on Pinterest (see my boards on The WHOLESTIC Method):

Happiness is a choice, not a result. Nothing will make you happy until you choose to be happy. No person will make you happy unless you decide to be happy. Your happiness will not come to you. It can only come from you.

A quote from an amazing friend to many...

I say my only wish is each of you finds peace in your heart, the joys of friendship, the love of family and the compassion for one another. Life's glass should always remain half full or at minimum a beautiful glass. Someone recently asked me about happiness. I'm certain it's quite different for each of us. I thought about it for a minute and realized the only way to *find happiness and sustain it is to **start by loving and accepting yourself**. By doing so, you can embrace the world and eliminate all which holds you down. Thanks again for allowing me to be a part of your lives. You make me smile. Please pray for a peaceful world and act only with kindness. Redemption and forgiveness... for we are all human.*

With that, I will end our overview of The WHOLESTIC Method eight elements to help improve the WHOLE you from the inside out. Who knows, maybe you are someone who should start with finding happiness first and go from there.

Now, let's move to The WHOLESTIC Method Roadmap Journal to figure out which element you need to start working on first and I encourage you to read my book, *Life is Not a Race*, to learn from my experience that more is not better.

Keep in mind that less is more. The more we do, the more risk for creating toxicity, but if we do little, then we risk the chance of creating deficiencies in our lives. Make sure you are being more mindful and putting more deposits into your wellness bank account.

Find that delicate balance between doing too much and doing too little. Look in the mirror each morning and say I love you, you matter, you are beautiful. Be grateful for what you have and send off good vibes. The changes will be subtle and yet quite noticeable.

Good luck.

The big five WHOLESTIC Method happiness tips for becoming a fat burner:
1. _____
2. _____
3. _____
4. _____
5. _____

The WHOLESTIC Method to improving fat loss, health, and performance for life and sports by working from the inside out.

Thank you for joining me on this new journey of living life as a journey and not as a race with The WHOLESTIC Method. Improve the whole you from the inside out and discover how amazing you feel. Now, get The WHOLESTIC Method workbook and start becoming a metabolically efficient, fat burning, fat-adapted-machine. You will be amazed by how much better you will look and feel when you teach your body to burn fat for fuel and reduce stress. Everyone's body system works more effectively and efficiently, plus you will feel better (happier) on the inside and out. First, we must do a few inner "core" exercises to individualize your journey. It is time to go deep and start learning about who you are – and what moves your soul. So, get your mind right.

Next step: on to your workbook.

LESSONS LEARNED FROM
THE WHOLE ATHLETE PODCAST

From my previous podcast called FIT FAT FAST (metabolic efficiency), to my current one, *The WHOLE Athlete*, we talk a lot about fueling, training, and performing for endurance sports such as Ironman Triathlons, marathons, and 50K trail running, as well as optimal health for all levels of athletes. I have learned a tremendous amount of information over the years, and I'm happy to share the most important of it with you.

TIM NOAKES

I have been fortunate to interview Professor Tim Noakes, OMS, MD, DSc, Ph.D. (hc) at the University of Cape Town and the Sports Science Institute of South Africa. Despite being an endurance athlete and closely following a prudent diet, Tim developed diabetes. Frustrated at his declining health and increased running times, he decided to switch to a high-fat, low carbohydrate diet as recommended by research from colleagues in North America.

The results astounded him as he could control his symptoms doing the exact opposite of the conventional medical approach. After sharing this experience, he faced a barrage of criticism concerning the lack of large-scale scientific trials to justify insulin-resistant/glucose-intolerant individuals following what became known as "The Tim Noakes Diet." In response, Tim has launched his foundation which intends to address the research gap into low-carb nutrition, thereby supporting healthier eating research. His foundation is registered and is applying for Non-Profit Corporation status with SARS.

Professor Noakes experimented, as Dr. Peter Attia (www.eatingacademy.com), with fasting during long workouts. Do we really need all of the processed energy foods for keeping us fueled up throughout workouts? Do we need to trust the major companies who claim that we need to eat and drink so much per hour when we exercise in order to keep our metabolism up?

In The WHOLESTIC Method program, we are eating real food, not boxed cereals, processed energy bars, or packaged crackers with ingredient lists that have words you can't pronounce. Professor Noakes is an excellent person to learn from about signs, like mood swings, of carbohydrate resistance. We can improve our performance for life and endurance sports on a lower carbohydrate and higher fat meal plan as we discover how many carbohydrates we are really consuming per day. Do you want to be a carbohydrate burner (glucose) or fat adapted (fat burning machine)? We have continuous energy if we are a fat burner but limited supply of energy if we are sugar burners. Carbohydrate metabolism involves the hormone insulin as we have discussed throughout the manual: excess carbs = stored fat.

This new way of eating (ancestral health is not new) is a lifestyle, not a diet. Learn the mantra now and repeat it every day. For best results, Professor Noakes expressed the need to make food and meal prep time a priority. Eating on the run and at restaurants is guaranteed to keep you eating high carbohydrates, sugar, grains, and the wrong type of oils.

I recommend reading Professor Noakes' book on *Banting and The Real Meal Revolution* he has started in South Africa. It explains what we have discussed: what are we designed to eat?

Banting merely discovered what human beings were designed to eat: what early humans ate 200,000 years ago. Respected biologists, geneticists, paleoanthropologists and theorists believe that human genes have hardly changed since human beings began their journey on earth. If you could put the entire human history into one day, we have only been eating cereals and grains for five minutes and sugar for five seconds, a very short amount of time in our existence. After the success experienced by William Banting on this low-carb, high-fat eating plan, the Banting diet became the standard treatment for weight loss in all major European and North American medical schools. But, in 1959, it was excluded from all the major medical and nutritional textbooks.

Professor Noakes and The Real Meal Revolution book provide interesting research and facts that validate our entire chapter on nutrition in The WHOLESTIC Method approach to fat loss, health, and performance.

"A common misconception in our society (world) is that eating fat, especially saturated fat, is bad for you and that it is a primary cause of high blood pressure, heart disease, and obesity. This is simply not true and was based on a flawed study by Ancel Keys in 1953. The truth is that a diet high in carbohydrates, particularly refined carbohydrates, and sugar are the cause of obesity, diabetes as well as other chronic illnesses. Vegetable (seed) oils and their derivatives such as margarine are also a contributing factor to heart disease, although manufacturers tell us the exact opposite."

As we continue to debate whether or not we need carbohydrates to survive, Professor Noakes is on a mission to teach us all not to be afraid of consuming healthy fats in our food plan.

This might come as a surprise, but of the three macronutrients in our diet (protein, fat, and carbohydrates), only carbohydrates are non-essential for human life. We cannot function properly for more than a few days without eating fat; without an adequate protein intake, we develop protein-calorie malnutrition within a few months. But avoiding carbohydrate has no short- or long-

term effects on humans, other than the (usually beneficial) effect of weight loss, especially in those who are the most overweight. While we need a constant supply of glucose, it can be produced by the liver from fat and protein and doesn't need to be ingested as carbohydrate in our diets.

Professor Noakes also wants to educate our bust the myth on cholesterol…

There is much evidence to support the fact that cholesterol is not the culprit in heart disease. A bit like a policeman g at the scene of the crime being blamed for the crime – cholesterol will only adhere to a 'leaking' artery wall which is damaged by inflammation – to protect you. By living on carbs and sugar those arteries remain inflamed. Sugar is the most inflammatory thing you can put into your mouth and will continue to rob you of perfect health. Grains are turned into sugar by the body. So a high carbohydrate diet will always foster inflammation in the body, not only in the arteries but the brain, liver, digestive tract and joints leading to many of the chronic diseases we see today which is supposedly 'incurable.' Many people report relief from all the above in a relatively short time after adopting the Banting lifestyle.

DINA GRIFFIN

A huge contribution to becoming a better fat burner starts with daily nutrition patterns (not just what you eat before, during, and after exercise). It all comes down to learning how to put together foods together that stabilize blood sugar levels. By controlling blood sugar and insulin levels, there are various cellular adaptations that occur to enable enhanced fat burning. Proper aerobic training certainly makes a difference in how well the body can burn fat, but we now know daily nutrition patterns have a significant influence.

I have interviewed Dina Griffin of eNRGperformance.com about her views on metabolism, diet, and becoming a fat burning machine. Dina is a Board Certified Specialist in Sports Dietetics, Certified Level II Metabolic Efficiency Training Specialist, and the eNRG performance Education Coordinator in Colorado.

There has always been a real emphasis on eating a huge amount of carbs as a necessary part of training and the general diet in the US. Dina says this is not a necessary step to take if you are able to make your metabolism burn fat instead of carbs. However, the way nutrition is taught to everyone, including athletes, it has been assumed that carbs are the way to go. Remember the old saying, "Carbo-load the night before a race?"

Instead, the approach to diet needs to be individualized. She is very cautious about a fasting approach. Men respond better to fasting than women, but she is reluctant to recommend fasting without a good reason. On the other hand, if, like me, you find yourself fasting by accident simply because you aren't hungry, that isn't really a problem. You aren't trying to follow an arbitrary schedule, rather you're listening to your body.

Dina also talks about ketosis and the need for more understanding of it. Again, diet is a matter of individual needs, but because the ketosis diet is extreme, it will require a greater degree of knowledge and education to identify carbs that might be hiding in foods generally thought of as fat or protein. In the end, she doesn't necessarily recommend one kind of diet, but you might do low carb instead of ketosis. The important thing is diet has to fit the individual and their needs.

If we eat right for our metabolic type or periodization plates and build up the aerobic engine by training by heart rate (get tested to determine your training zones to burn fat for fuel) during our training workouts, we can improve our metabolic efficiency or rather the ability to burn more fat and improve mighty mitochondria. The mitochondria are part of the cell to generate energy or ATP; fat oxidation occurs in the cells so we want more mitochondria to become more efficient fat burners.

Why do we need to burn fat besides the obvious: the more efficient we are at burning fat for fuel in training and racing, then the fewer calories we need to consume, less GI stress, and inflammation. Our endurance training puts lots of stress on our body and increases our inflammatory markers: adrenal response, sex hormones, hormone levels, and blood sugar levels. By becoming less reliant on carbohydrates for fuel, we improve our blood sugar levels and more benefits.

If we train hard and consume high carbohydrate diet, we are constantly creating inflammation in our body. Our classic refueling foods are processed and lack nutrient density. We want to eat a real food anti-inflammatory plan instead of the high carb, processed factory-made foods that cause us to stay on the blood sugar roller coaster and overeat. We don't need 300-400 calories per hour for long distance training and racing if you are a metabolic efficient athlete, fewer calories are needed if you are burning fat as your main fuel source. The amount of carbs varies person to person as well as your training phase. The goal is to balance your blood sugar levels to burn fat, not necessarily be in ketosis or be extremely low-carb to be a metabolic efficient fat burning machine.

Do you know how many carbs you eat per day?

The traditional approach to diet during training has emphasized the consumption of carbs, and it has generally been assumed the only source of energy for the body is through carbohydrates.

Dina points out you can teach the body to become a fat burning machine, and that there are many more calories stored in fat than in the body's limited stores of carbs.

Dina also discusses whether a high-intensity training approach is better than the long, slow endurance sessions that have been the norm. Again, the better option is a middle ground rather than an all-or-nothing approach. Athletes generally do too much HIIT or too much endurance training. What's important is to balance those kinds of workout, the same way you balance carbs with fat in your diet.

Check out our past episodes on Metabolic Efficiency with Dina from ENRG Performance on The WHOLE Athlete podcast.

JILL GRUNEWALD

What about the fear of fat, cholesterol, and heart disease?

Jill Grunewald from www.healthfulelements.com was my guest co-host to talk about the fear of fat, hormones, cholesterol, and heart disease myths. Jill loves to talk about the importance of dietary fat and the fear of fat. Concerns people have about eating fat, getting fatter, and heart disease are never ending and we need to point out some facts or rather bust some myths.

The nutritional myth that saturated fat is bad for us started with a flawed study by Ancel Keys which lead to the years of low-fat/non-fat and high carbohydrate (usually refined, processed, and filled with sugar). Beginning in the 1940s, Ancel Keys, known as a pioneering American physiologist, helped establish the link between cholesterol and cardiovascular disease which started the fear of fat, cholesterol, and saturated fat. Ancel hypothesized that saturated fat in the diet is unhealthy and should be avoided. His hypothesis was a little incorrect.

Our high carb-low fat processed foods diet is known as the Standard American Diet – or S.A.D. Perhaps, our fear of fat has led us to an increase in auto-immune disorders, inflammation, and disease, as well as a hormonal train wreck.

Jill talks about how our low-fat diet creates a mess with our hormones, but we continue to have this fear of fat stuck in our heads. We need to look at what types of fats are bad such as manufactured fats. Good fats include, as you should know by now, quality sources of fat egg yolks, fatty fish, avocados, Ghee, grass-fed butter, and healthy oils such as coconut, olive oil, and avocado oils.

The fear of cholesterol is ingrained in our heads. People are still going for the egg whites to avoid the yolks that are filled with nutritious essential fat-soluble vitamins. A diet high in sugar may be what raises our risk for heart disease by promoting metabolic syndrome. Metabolic syndrome is a combination of red flags: high blood pressure, high insulin, leptin resistance, high triglycerides, liver dysfunction, and visceral fat accumulation.

Actually, cholesterol heals damaged cells, anti-inflammatory, and—don't kill the messenger—cholesterol comes to the rescue many times. We have gotten mixed messages on what is bad or good cholesterol as well as what are acceptable cholesterol blood work results... what is high and low cholesterol? Does high cholesterol equal increased risk for heart disease? You may want to dig deeper into this theory by reading Jimmy Moore's book, *Cholesterol Clarity - What the HDL?*

Did you know that even hypothyroidism can lead to high cholesterol? Jill talks in our podcast (search on www.thewholeathletepodcast.com) about the relationship of hormones and cholesterol (king of the chart), the importance of Pregnenolone, the flowchart of the hormones (see references) and how they communicate. Some hormones make other hormones such as pregnenolone. Cholesterol is the king of the throne, followed by pregnenolone. If one is disrupted, we have a domino effect in the body, as I discuss in my book, *Life is Not a Race.*

Everything is connected and—big shocker—imbalances may be related to low-fat diets we started twenty to thirty years ago. We should not be afraid of healthy fats as eating good fats helps you lose fat - metabolic burner. We have been trained to believe eating fat-free, processed, low-calorie foods help us lose weight. Just the opposite is true. Not getting enough fat can make you metabolically stagnant and lower your metabolism. Fat is a fuel for our bodies and gives us long-lasting fuel for energy. Saturated fats help reduce bloating by regulating salt retention ratio.

If you read my book, you will find out how quickly I gained weight around my belly (and everywhere) once my HPA Axis – adrenal dysfunction occurred. My cortisol was completely out of control (or HPA Axis dysregulation) which led to my accumulation of belly fat. Thyroid and adrenals are fat dependent to operate properly. More reasons to eat fat and not fear getting fat... eat sugar if you want to get fat.

Did you know to improve Vitamin D absorption you should take it with a meal with fat to absorb the best? Another factoid is your brain function is two-thirds fat which is why brain neurological disorders do well on a ketogenic diet. There is a link with dementia and lack of fat as well as other brain-related diseases as we discussed in the ketosis section.

To regulate blood sugar and release of it into the bloodstream, avoid hyperglycemia and hypoglycemic blood sugar roller coaster = inflammation and more negative effects in the body.

Jill reminds us to sidestep bad fats as seed oils, hydrogenated soybean oil, trans fats which are actually fake processed fats created in a lab. Instead, go for the grass-fed dairy and meat instead of processed and pasteurized dairy. Our hormones regulate everything in our body. Fat and cholesterol are the building blocks of hormones. Without healthy sources of fat, you will eventually have health problems.

Find out about three-month coaching plans with Jill via www.healthfulelements.com.

Other sources:

http://tinyurl.com/WrongAboutSatFat

http://tinyurl.com/CholesterolBodyHealth

http://tinyurl.com/HormonePathways

http://tinyurl.com/AncelKeysWiki

http://tinyurl.com/SatFatHrtDisease

JIMMY MOORE

I interviewed author Jimmy Moore (http://www.livinlavidalowcarb.com) on how to use good fats and the importance of eliminating the abundance of carbohydrates in our diet. Jimmy lost 180 pounds and his approaches to dieting have been called radical though he points out his prior diet was as radical in the other direction.

Jimmy talks about the benefits of eating good fat and other aspects of diet, including a discussion what seems to be a common misconception that the American food system is the best in the world. Jimmy traveled in Europe and extols the virtues of something called double cream. This is a delicious, thick, dairy product that puts all other attempts at creaminess to shame.

He describes the importance of recognizing that Type 2 diabetes needs to be recognized as carb intolerance. He questions the value of giving people drugs before there has been any attempt to modify diet which is the root of the problem. In his words, insulin has definitely been a help to Type 1 sufferers, but for Type 2 patients, it has simply become a way to cover the bad dietary choices required by common misconceptions about nutrition, which generally include a large number of carbs.

Check out this video where Jimmy talks about canola oil:

https://youtu.be/omjWmLG0EAs

The WHOLESTIC Method Manual & Workbook

Even though it's completely pro-canola, it can't help but educate people about how the oil is actually made.

Jimmy and co-author, Maria Emmerich, have the *Ketogenic Cookbook* available so you can easily enjoy creative, low-carb recipes and goodies. Jimmy is also the author of two more books with Dr. Eric Westman, *Keto Clarity* (http://tinyurl.com/KetoClarity) and *Cholesterol Clarity* (http://tinyurl.com/CholesterolClarity) and one more coming on *Intermittent Fasting*.

Jimmy Moore talks about how what we eat increases inflammation in our body. Inflammation is raised by our (over) consumption of refined carbohydrates and man-made vegetable oils as canola oil, seed oil, etc. We should test the specific number of LCL particle size. Statin drugs have so many side effects and often unnecessary since most people are prescribed statin drugs based on lab tests that are not looking at the big picture of inflammatory markers and the root cause. Jimmy says high cholesterol itself is not a disease and many myths are associated with getting high cholesterol. Once again, it is the sugar in our foods that is the real culprit of inflammation. Chronic health problems are tied to poor nutrition in our culture as we are addicted to sugar and quick, easily prepared foods. To lower the risk of heart disease, eat real foods that are anti-inflammatory.

Also, as with my entire The WHOLESTIC Method elements, excessive and constant stress, as well as the lack of sleep, can also raise inflammation.

Are you putting all of these together?

Saturated fat is **not** inflammatory. Think about coconut oil. Consume lots of organic (ideally) green leafy vegetables and non-starchy carbohydrates along with higher healthy fats and moderate clean protein (grass fed, free range).

Do you see a pattern or a rather common theme?

Blood lab tests should measure inflammatory markers in the body and include LDL particle test, triglycerides, and C - reactive protein per Jimmy Moore.

- HDL >50
- Triglycerides<100
- HDL<50
- Triglycerides>100
- Blood sugar =>140 too high, too many carbohydrates
- LDL should be below 70 mg/dl
- HDL should be below 40mg/dl (men), 50 mg/dl (women)
- The HSCRP test for inflammation, number under 3. 0 is good, less than 1. 0 is optimal

Cholesterol is carried in lipoprotein throughout the body to it can be delivered to its job site to perform its essential responsibilities as:

- Maintains the structure of cells and vessels to improve our overall health and function in the body
- Precursor to important hormones in our body as testosterone, estrogen, androgen, and progesterone
- Precursor to corticosteroids that play a role in protecting the body against stress and disease (cortisol and DHEA)
- Used as insulation around nerves to help promote healthy nervous system function
- Helps prevent diseases in the nervous system
- Essential for brain function
- Aids in digestive system since bile salts are made from cholesterol
- Helps strengthen the intestinal walls in the digestion system
- The precursor to Vitamin D which is an important nutrient for supporting our immune, nervous, and reproduction system as well as insulin production and mineral metabolism.
- Improves serotonin receptors in the brain – which the serotonin neurotransmitter provides a feeling of well-being and low levels of serotonin are, connect to depression.

Source: http://tinyurl.com/CholesterolBodyHealth2

Recommended reading:

Fallon, Sally, and Enig, Mary. (1999) Nourishing Traditions: The Cookbook that Challenges Politically Correct Nutrition and the Diet Dictocrats.

Schwarzbein, Diana. (1999) The Schwarzbein Principle: The Truth About Losing Weight, Being Healthy, and Feeling Younger.

http://www.cholesterolclarity.com/

Learn more about the benefits of Ketosis for the brain and more benefits...
MCT oil, Coconut Oil, and Ketosis:

www.mariamindbodyhealth.com
http://www.dietdoctor.com/low-carb/keto#intro
http://tinyurl.com/VeryLowCarbDiet
http://tinyurl.com/YourBrainKetones
www.livinlavidalowcarb.com
www.cholesterolclarity.com
https://authoritynutrition.com/mct-oil-101/
http://draxe.com/caprylic-acid/
http://www.coconutketones.com/whatifcure.pdf
http://www.coconutketones.com/
http://draxe.com/mct-oil/

DR. JOEL ROSEN

What about Ketogenic Diet for those with Adrenal Issues – stress disease?

I came across Dr. Joel Rosen's blogs online, and I was interested in learning more about his personal story of adrenal fatigue and recovery which was similar to my story. When I was in the beginning stages of adrenal exhaustion, I was unable to tolerate any sugar (including fruit) without spiking my blood sugar levels sky high and a headache within seconds.

If our adrenals are broken, we may struggle with regulating our blood sugar levels so ketosis may be an ideal solution for those recovering from adrenal fatigue. We need to find the right amount of dietary fats, proteins, and carbs to find the right balance for you to be in ketosis. If you get the shakes and light headed if you don't have a meal or want to crash after eating, you may have cortisol levels responding to the stressor.

We often get stuck in the chronic stress roller coaster... over and over again which results in chronic adrenal fatigue. Then, we become maladaptive in responding to cortisol = acute, maladaptive chronic phase. We can't regulate blood sugar levels throughout the day, and then we are asked to eat multiple meals and snacks throughout the day to manage the blood sugar. If we are stuck in the adrenal fatigue state, our cortisol levels are not functioning correctly. We have too many stress triggers, so we need to decrease the stress alerts by switching to ketosis.

How should we eat if you have adrenal fatigue? Eat when hungry, but measure your glucose and ketones in the morning once you understand your values — ketones .5- 3. 0 and glucose 60-80.

Once in the more ketogenic zone and relate it to your hunger. Do you need to fuel up based on your numbers? Listen to your body if you don't measure your ketones and glucose.

Another treatment method Dr. Rosen offers at his Boca Health clinic is improving the brain function. Listen to his explanation of the brain therapy:

Improvements we can implement...

1. Breathing - posture
2. Adequate hydration with healthy water
3. Healthy proteins, fats, and carbs with not too much sugar
4. Reduce stimulant use such as caffeine and supplements for energy
5. Proper supplementation based on your weak links and what response they are having with your body... we don't need them every day if feeling good

Source: www.bocahealthcenter.com or www.adrenalsociety.com for opt-in on the X-Factor on what is missing on adrenal fatigue treatment

DR. EDWARDS

I did a similar podcast with Dr. Edwards who is a D. O. and discovered over his years working with athletes that he needed to treat their health and differently as telling athletes not to do something is not an effective solution. Dr. Edwards started to look at the big picture as he realized the traditional treatments didn't always work for everyone. He strives to optimize health and their human performance with his unique treatment system - the integrated approach as I love as well.

Dr. Edwards' mission when working with clients created the foundational approach the Healthy Trinity for his intervention and treatment plan based on his experience: Exercise and Nutrition then the three R's... similar to The WHOLESTIC Method Approach...

1. Rest
2. Recovery from exercise
3. Reducing Stress

When those three R's go haywire, medical problems and our health are comprised. As I love to say, we need to work from the inside out to be the healthiest versions of ourselves to lose weight, eliminate inflammation, and reduce the risk of diseases. Are we eating for our right metabolic type? The way to treat clients or how to eat is not one size fits all, but we all start the same. Eat real food such as recommended in the Paleo Diet.

Dr. Edwards starts most clients on the Paleo diet or Primal Paleo to help them improve gut issues, food sensitivities, inflammation and more. A generalized Paleo type of diet is a good intro. We both like to think of this of the real food plan and not using the Paleo manufactured processed foods on the market. The term has gotten blown up in the food marketing industry. The word Paleo is a natural food plan as we were designed to eat. A natural eating plan - minimally invasive and limited intervention in the food is consuming.

The mainstream media confuses all of us what to eat, but really we need to look at the source of our food products. Are they farm raised? Organic? Free Range? Non-GMO? To eat meat or not to eat meat. This is why we have a podcast... to clear up the confusion.

What supplements do you need to add to your food plan? Even if we eat real food, we still need to supplement our diet with an additional source of nutrients such as Omega-3. We want Omega 6 in balance with Omega-3 fatty acids, or else we create inflammation in our body. The problem is in the balance of the two ...we don't all need a fish oil supplement but our SAD has way too much Omega-6 pro-inflammatory fatty acids. We need both omega 3 and omega 6 but in balance. Yin and Yang. Balance in the nervous system.

Chronic inflammation is common in many people that we can improve with nutrition. Then, the cholesterol and thyroid issues... why do we hear about so many people taking medication for problems they could improve or get to the root cause then improve the function? Maybe we have toxins or nutritional deficiencies in our body. How do we know?

Get testing information available for free at www.fitnessforwardstudio.com/ lab testing or find the Spectra cell lab test Dr. Edwards suggest to test why a client feels the way they feel. Look at the WHOLE picture.

Do we need to take statin drugs? What is the updated literature state? Or, do Doctors not have time to research and rely on the pharmaceutical drug reps for updates in research that supports medication. What about the side effects of the medication?

What about gut health? Do we need probiotics? We have different strains of bacteria naturally in our gut. Look for a probiotic that is a strain that is identified and studied to interact with the human gut. I use Dr. Pearlmutter's Probiotics, or you can order various ones on my website www.fitnessforwardstudio.com/ supplements.

We want to test the gut and digestive system with lab testing to test for infections, yeast or candida type of infections or parasites. I had a few tests conducted the last three years with the Kalish Method and Christopher Kelly to find out my parasite infection I was not aware of. We need a healthy gut so look for lab testing if you have any symptoms... check your bowel movement each day.

VINNIE TORTORICH

Vinnie has been a personal trainer to Hollywood for years transforming bodies with their exercise routine and nutrition. His secret for helping his celebrity clients cut fat and get lean quickly to look amazing is simple, but it's also challenging for most people who are addicted to sugar. Vinnie coaches his clients and writes in his book about the No Sugar No Grains (NSNG) eating guidelines for losing weight and feeling great. If you want to speed up fat loss and improve health for optimal performance, then drop the sugar and the grains.

Everyone wants instant results and the quick fix solution. They all want to be fit, lean, and healthy right now. To get lasting results, we need to change the mindset that avoiding sugar and grains is a long-term lifestyle change. Yes, you will see and feel the changes after sticking with a real food plan without sugar and grains as you will end up eating real food instead of processed empty calorie foods.

Vinnie shares his personal story and battle with cancer in his book *Fitness Confidential* about eliminating sugar to starve cancer. His doctor told him to stay away from sugar as she was learning about how cancer cells feed on sugar. Since grains play a similar role as sugar in the body, Vinnie decided to practice twenty-five years of his own advice. Vinnie has been following his own NSNG protocol to avoid cancer, but also to help his performance in ultra-cycling events he has completed in the past. Since he continues to win the battle against cancer, Vinnie follows a ketogenic diet to keep his cancer in remission. Vinnie doesn't promote the ketogenic diet for his own clients as it is not necessary for them to be fat–adapted. If you follow a no sugar no grain food plan, you will most likely teach your body to burn fat for fuel. You don't need to be in ketosis unless, as we discussed, you are fighting cancer, neurological disorders, or severe weight management issues. Vinnie continues to keep his Leukemia in remission with the way he lives, trains, and eats. You don't need to be in dietary ketosis to make NSNG work to help you burn fat and lose weight. Don't worry... as more research continues to come out, we will do podcast episodes on this topic in the future.

Keeping it simple... avoid sugar and grains if you want to improve fat loss, health, and performance. Vinnie talks about in his book to focus on eating real food especially non-processed real foods. To eat NSNG, focus on eating vegetables, fruits, nuts/seeds, legumes, healthy fats, and meats.

We have talked a lot about why we need to break the sugar addiction and how it impacts your health, including the fat storing hormone insulin but why avoid grains?

Grains have a similar effect on the body as sugar so eliminate sugar and grains for at least thirty days to find out how you feel. According to the USDA, grains are any food made from wheat, rice, oats, cornmeal, barley, or another cereal grain is a grain product. Bread, pasta, oatmeal, breakfast cereals, tortillas, and grits are examples of grain products.

Vinnie is not a fan of eating quinoa because it is a grain, which means it is not an NSNG food. Quinoa is definitely on the do not eat list according to Vinnie's NSNG program. More detailed information on grains can be found at: http://www.choosemyplate.gov/food-groups/grains.html.

What do people eat when following a food plan that doesn't include sugar or grains? Simple. NSNG snack options include low glycemic fruit, cut veggies, hard boiled eggs, beef jerky, full-fat cheese, raw nuts, olives, pumpkin seeds, eighty-five percent (85%) or greater dark chocolate, deviled eggs (homemade mayo), pepperoni slices, coconut oil, avocado, lettuce rolled up with smoked salmon and full fat cream cheese, hummus and celery, pickles, tofu, shot of olive oil, coffee with heavy cream (or grass-fed butter or coconut oil).

As we know, most people get moody and angry if they are on the blood sugar roller coaster and it is not fun to spend time with unhappy people. We are happy if we eat real whole foods... keep it simple as Vinnie says to his clients and just avoid sugar and grains.

WILLIAM WOLCOTT

One of my favorite books is by William L. Wolcott, *The Metabolic Typing Diet* (Doubleday, 2000) - which we talk a lot about in my coaching program to get people eating right for their type of metabolism. I was fortunate to chat with Bill Wolcott, the founder of Metabolic Typing and an advocate of the individual approach to diet. Instead of believing certain foods are good and certain foods are bad, Bill has found from practicing Metabolic Typing for over nearly forty years that foods are good or bad for you depending on how your body uses food, not on intrinsic properties of the food itself.

While some types will respond best to a diet of higher protein and fat, others may respond well to a higher percentage of carbohydrates. This depends on the metabolism of the person involved. That's why a given diet will cause some people to lose weight, have no effect on others, but actually cause a third group to gain weight. Likewise, some Metabolic Types will lower cholesterol on a low protein and fat, high carb diet while others find that their cholesterol goes up on that diet. And, certain other types find that a high protein and high-fat diet relative to carb intake lowers cholesterol, but that same diet raises it in others.

This notion of treating the person who has the disease over the disease that has the person is not new but rather was a common theme in every ancient system of medicine, e.g., Ayurveda, Chinese, Egyptian, Greek, etc., and has been overlooked in the drug-oriented orthodox system of our modern era. Unfortunately, neglecting diet has a cost; the skyrocketing statistics of degenerative conditions throughout modern societies. Degenerative disease and sub-clinical health complaints have become so common that having such is the norm. But, Metabolic Typing has revealed that is not normal at all. Rather, the body is designed to function perfectly, and it's largely through failing to meet genetically-based requirements of one's Metabolic Type that our health becomes compromised. There has never been and there never will be one diet that is right for everyone. The only diet that is right for you is the one that is right for YOUR Metabolic Type.

Here are just a few keynotes from our podcast discussion:

- Any MT can be a fat burner or a sugar burner, depending on how efficient their metabolism is functioning – that's in terms of normal versus overweight. That said, note that Fast Oxidizers (FOs) are overly-reliant on an extremely efficient in burning carbs and that's why they do well on higher protein and fat diets to balance out their fast oxidation rates. That is not a bad thing for healthy FOs. They are also, of course, efficient at burning fat. The issue is problematic when a metabolism can only burn sugars and can't burn fats very well.
- Allergies/sensitivities have nothing to do with Metabolic Type (MT). Any MT can develop an allergy (aberration) to any food by eating a diet wrong for his Metabolic Type.
- There is no such thing as a Paleo Diet that is right for everyone. Think Weston Price. There is a different Paleo diet for different geographies and climates. Or said differently, there are different Paleo diets for different Metabolic Types. The Eskimo/Inuit ate all protein and fat and almost no carbohydrate, and the Tukasenta ate over ninety percent (90%) carbs and only ten percent (10%) proteins and fats, yet both indigenous cultures were perfectly healthy and virtually free of degenerative disease.

- Ketogenic is a therapeutic diet only – not a lifetime, healthy diet. It is an imbalanced state and not the normal, healthy state for any MT. Slow Oxidizers (SOs), however, have a greater propensity for it as compared to FOs since they burn carbs too slowly. Decreasing carbs and increasing fats and proteins can quickly shift their metabolisms ketogenic. That's why in terms of maximizing cellular energy production from the diet, they do best on lower protein and fats and higher carbohydrate diets.

The big five WHOLESTIC Lessons for becoming a fat burner:

1. _____
2. _____
3. _____
4. _____
5. _____

Don't forget that in order to improve fat loss, health and performance you must work on all of The WHOLESTIC Method elements. Start by improving nutrition first, then work on improving the other eight elements; then you will reset your body to become a fat burner – not a sugar burner and be a happier person.

See more on my free gift download on www.debbiepotts.net.

PART TWO

The WHOLESTIC
Method Workbook

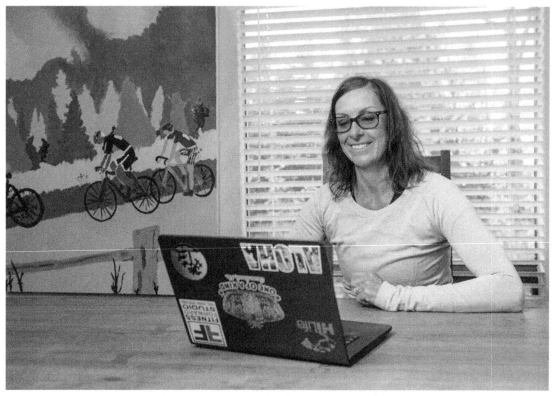

A Program designed to
Transform the WHOLE You
from the Inside Out

Burn Fat-Optimize Health-Improve Performance

LIFE IS NOT A RACE IT IS A JOURNEY PACE THE WHOLE YOU FROM THE INSIDE OUT

WITH THE WHOLESTIC METHOD

STOP. PAUSE. RESET. RECALIIBRATE. SLOW DOWN. ENJOY THE JOURNEY. BREATHE. HUM. SING. NO RUSH. RECHARGE. UNPLUG. DISCONNECT. RECONNECT. REST. SMILE. LAUGH. HUG. LOVE LIFE. LET IT GO.

Transform the WHOLE You
Contact Debbie Potts to learn how!
www.thewholeathletepodcast.com

TABLE OF CONTENTS

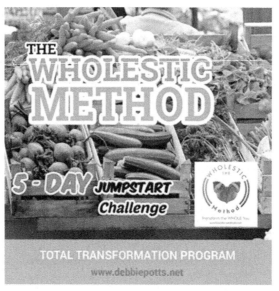

THE WORKBOOK INTRO

A re you ready for a change and to transform the WHOLE you?

Are you ready to feel and look better... on the inside and out?

Let's get started on The WHOLESTIC Method program. Hopefully, you just finished reading The WHOLESTIC Method manual and are ready to transform the WHOLE you. The workbook is your roadmap to transforming your body and mind.

We are going to train the WHOLE you to become a more efficient fat burner, a health optimizer, and improve your performance in life and sports. To get there, we need to figure out where we are now before we figure out where we are headed by working from the inside out. We then look at your why and then move on to the roadmap questions and lifestyle questionnaires.

Phase One is the 5-Day Jumpstart Challenge to prepare you for the new eating and lifestyle habits. Then, we move to Phase Two, the 21-Day Sugar Detox and Reset Challenge to help you work on make commitments to our established goals and our "areas of opportunities." Finally, Phase Three is our ongoing lifestyle program to help you stay on track and committed to The WHOLESTIC Method way of living life.

Often, we start a new fitness program, a new diet, or a new type of detox challenge without having a plan, a roadmap, or, more importantly, learning about ourselves from the inside and out. Before you commit to The WHOLESTIC Method transformational program, we need to peel off a few layers so we can discover your personality, dreams, goals, challenges, obstacle, and areas of opportunity. We will create an inner roadmap then move to the eight elements of The WHOLESTIC Method.

Discover your WHY by digging deeply to get clarity and vision on your life roadmap. Block at least an hour to answer these questions and maybe take a break to go for a walk or bike ride to get more precision on your responses. Sometimes, it helps to take time out to create a plan to decide which road you want to take in life. Where is your journey taking you? Visualization helps to get on the road you set out to take as you get a clearer picture and define what you want to do in life or achieve... and why.

Now, go find a quiet, peaceful spot to allow your creative brain to emerge. Let the ideas flow. I love to write outside in my backyard, in my home office, or take notes after a bike ride or while on an airplane. Find your happy place where your mind is clear and you can get in the deep zone. Getting clarity in your goals will help you determine how to create a daily, weekly, monthly, quarterly, and annual roadmap to improve the WHOLE you from the inside out. You will improve your performance in all areas of life if you take the time to find out where you are headed and why.

We need to stop the glorification of being busy and racing through the day. Learn how to recalibrate your life so you can achieve your fat loss, health, and performance goals.

Our first step is getting you to discover your values, your vision and what you want your legacy you want to leave in life. Why am I asking you to work from the inside out to improve your ability to burn fat, to optimize your health, and/or to improve your performance in sports? Well, I have discovered from my own experiences and from my mentors that we need to stop and reflect on our purpose to determine our "why" in order to grow personally, professionally, mentally, and physically.

If you don't know where you are going, then how are you going to get there?

It is time to make yourself a priority and focus on getting connected to yourself and doing some "inner core" work by following the following steps here in this workbook:

- Step #1 – Finding Your Why
- Step #2 – THE WHOLESTIC Method Roadmap
- Step #3 – Working From The Inside Out To Transform The Whole You
- Step #4 – Phase One - The WHOLESTIC Method 5-Day Jumpstart Challenge
- Step #5 – Phase Two - The 21-Day Fat Loss And Reset Challenge
- Step #6 – Phase Three - The Maintenance Program
- Step #7 – Health Questionnaire And History

It is time to get your mind right to begin your new transformational journey – The WHOLESTIC Method.

"You are too concerned about what was and what will be. There is a saying: yesterday is history, tomorrow is a mystery, but today is a gift. That is why it is called the "present."
Shifu: [sighs] Yes, I know."
~Kung Fu Panda

STEP #1
FINDING YOUR WHY

The 5-Day Jumpstart Challenge and the 21-Day Fat Loss and Reset Challenge both require the right mindset, commitment, and motivation. Teamwork is also a key part in making these new changes.

What is your one love? One of my mentors, Paul Chek, influenced my questions...

1. *What is your motive to do the program?*
2. *What is your dream worth experiencing?*
3. *What do you love enough for a change?*

EXERCISE #1: THE WHOLE YOU QUESTIONNAIRE

Be sure to complete these questions before you start the Phase One program for best results.

READINESS QUESTIONNAIRE:

This is our prep time to help you become mentally prepared to make The WHOLESTIC Method lifestyle improvements to allow you to achieve your fat loss and health goals. Let's do some "inner core" work before we get any further. We want to get to the root cause of why we are where we are. Go deep as you write your answers to the questions in this next section.

I want you to ask yourself: why do you need to lose weight? Why are you stressed? Why are you not sleeping? Whatever your goals are, get to the core by going deeper and peeling one layer off at a time. We are going to discover more about you to lose weight, get healthy, or improve performance every day. However, we need to start working from the inside out. As I always tell clients, if you want to look and stay the same, then continue doing what you are doing now. If you want to create change and establish new healthy habits for life, we are going to need to push the "reset" button and switch up how we do a typical twenty-one-day sugar detox challenge.

The following questions will help determine your level of readiness to making lifestyle changes, your motivation toward reaching your goals, and identifying obstacles to your success of becoming a fat burning machine or just to feel your best and happier each day.

Remember, there are no right or wrong answers. The information you share will be used to help you and your coach create the best goals and program for you.

Let's take the WHOLESTIC approach to detoxing our body and start to reprogram our habits and mindset.

- Are you placing your health at risk because of your current behaviors or lifestyle? If so, please describe. (e.g. smoking, drug use, sedentary, overweight, etc.)

  _____

  _____

  _____

  _____

  _____

- Are you seeking to make lifetime changes or reach a short-term, temporary goal?

  _____

  _____

  _____

  _____

  _____

- Are you open to trying different approaches, or do you have preferred methods, areas to avoid, etc.?
  ❑ Yes   ❑ No   ❑ Maybe
  Explain: _____

  _____

  _____

  _____

  _____

- Are you willing to set realistic goals? Are you prepared to deal with possible setbacks?
  ❑ Yes   ❑ No   ❑ Maybe
  Explain: _____

  _____

  _____

  _____

  _____

- Are you willing to make lifestyle changes, or would you rather maintain your current lifestyle with slight modifications?

  ❑ Yes ❑ No ❑ Maybe

  Explain: _____

  _____

  _____

  _____

  _____

- Have you made previous attempts at lifestyle changes? If so, what were the results?

  ❑ Yes ❑ No ❑ Maybe

  Explain: _____

  _____

  _____

  _____

  _____

- Compared to previous attempts to lose weight, how motivated are you at this time to try to change your lifestyle? (On a scale of 1-5; 1 = not at all motivated, 5 = extremely motivated.)

  1   2   3   4   5

- Are there outside factors (work, family, travel, etc.) that could impact your ability to make lifestyle changes?

  ❑ Yes ❑ No ❑ Maybe

  If so, list: _____

  _____

  _____

  _____

  _____

- How confident are you that you can work regular exercise into your daily schedule starting tomorrow? (On a scale of 1-5; 1 = not at all confident, 5 = extremely confident.)

  1   2   3   4   5

- Indicate your busiest and easiest days of the week.

  Busiest: _____

  Easiest: _____

List any challenges that are as a result of your present situation (e.g. "none of my clothes fit," "I have no energy," "My blood pressure is too high.")

_____
_____
_____
_____
_____
_____

- Check the areas you're looking for improvements:
    Body Weight   _____
    Body Image and Appearance   _____
    Gut Health and Digestion   _____
    Fatigue and Energy   _____
    Athletic Performance   _____
    Injury Repair and Recovery   _____
    Other _____

Self-Image:

1. What is that one thing you could change in your life right now if you could?

_____
_____
_____
_____
_____

2. How do you see yourself from the outside? What do you look like?

_____
_____
_____
_____

3. What do you want to change about the way you look, if anything?

_____
_____
_____
_____
_____
_____

4. What type of diets have you been on in the past?

_____
_____
_____
_____
_____

5. How do you feel about your body weight or image of yourself?

_____
_____
_____
_____
_____

6. Do you have a realistic goal weight that would make you feel comfortable and happy?
   ❑ Yes   ❑ No   ❑ Maybe
   Explain: _____

_____
_____
_____
_____

Travel and Adventure:

1. Do you take vacation or "life" breaks to disconnect?
   ❑ Yes   ❑ No   ❑ Maybe
   Explain: _____

_____
_____

_____
_____
_____

2. What do you do to disconnect and unplug?

_____
_____
_____
_____
_____

3. How frequently do you take mini-vacations or days off just for yourself? Explain.

_____
_____
_____
_____
_____

4. What trips, experiences, or adventures are on your "bucket list?"

_____
_____
_____
_____

5. How could you carve out more time for vacations and breaks from the busyness of life?

_____
_____
_____
_____

Connection Time:

1. Do you take one day a week or more to "unplug" and stay off-line? If not, how could you make this a goal and a priority?

   ❑ Yes   ❑ No   ❑ Maybe

   Explain:

   _____

   _____

   _____

   _____

2. Do you set up specific times each day to check email and messages? If so, when? If not, make a plan on how prioritize your day and block off specific time for returning messages.

   ❑ Yes   ❑ No   ❑ Maybe

   Explain:

   _____

   _____

   _____

   _____

3. Do you use your phone or read your electronic device when you are...?

   ❑ Eating meals with friends or family?
   ❑ Driving your car?
   ❑ Exercising?
   ❑ Vacations?

   ...how can you change your habits?

   _____

   _____

THE EIGHT ELEMENTS OF THE WHOLESTIC METHOD QUESTIONNAIRE

Nutrition: Relationship with food and alcohol

1. Do you eat when bored, stressed, or lonely?

    ❑ Yes ❑ No ❑ Maybe

    If so, what is your why?

    _____

    _____

    _____

    _____

    _____

    _____

2. Do you crave sugary sweets and carbohydrates? Or salt?

    ❑ Yes ❑ No ❑ Maybe

    Why do you think you have these cravings?

    _____

    _____

    _____

    _____

3. Which foods do you have a challenge just eating one small bite? Which foods do you overeat or can't eat just one?

_____

_____

_____

_____

_____

4. How frequently to you dine out or pick up take out each week? If more than two times per week, is it because you don't like cooking, are short on time, or why?

_____

_____

_____

_____

_____

5. Do you drink alcohol to relax, unwind, or decompress?
    ❑ Yes   ❑ No   ❑ Maybe
    If so, why do you feel that alcohol as a glass of wine helps you unwind?

_____

_____

_____

_____

_____

6. Do you drink alcohol with dinner more than once per week?
    ❑ Yes   ❑ No   ❑ Maybe
    If so, how many glasses? Are you able to go through a meal without a glass?

_____

_____

_____

_____

7.   Do you ever test resting blood sugar levels in the morning?
     ❏ Yes   ❏ No
     a.   Would you be interested in testing your resting blood sugar levels for 30 days?
          ❏ Yes   ❏ No
     b.   Would you be interested in testing your blood sugar levels and/or ketones after eating?
          ❏ Yes   ❏ No
     c.   Would you measure your heart rate post meals to learn about food sensitivities?
          ❏ Yes   ❏ No

Exercise:
1.   Do you see yourself as an active person consistently? ❏ Yes   ❏ No   ❏ Maybe
     If not, why? _____

     _____

     _____

     _____

     _____

2.   Do you enjoy playing any specific sports or competing in events? What type of exercise do you enjoy and look forward to joining in?

     _____

     _____

     _____

3. Are you happy with your fitness level now?

❏ Yes ❏ No ❏ Maybe

Any areas for improvement you would like to focus on?

_____

_____

_____

_____

Please evaluate your status in the following:

   a. Strength? _____

   b. Endurance? _____

   c. Speed? _____

   d. Mobility? _____

   e. Stability and Balance? _____

4. In the next five years, what are your athletic or fitness goals?

_____

_____

_____

_____

5. Do you use any devices to track workout effort level?

   ❏ Heart rate monitor?

   ❏ Garmin watch?

   ❏ Strava?

   ❏ Apple Watch?

   ❏ Fitbit?

   ❏ Other: _____

Quality of Sleep:

1. Do you use your computer, phone, or iPad one hour or less before bedtime?

   ❏ Yes   ❏ No

2. How long does it take for you to fall asleep on average? _____

   _____

   How many hours do you sleep? _____

3. What time do you go to bed at night? _____

4. How many times do you wake up per night? _____

   _____

   Do you wake up in the middle of the night and can't fall back asleep?

   ❏ Yes   ❏ No

5. What time do you wake up in the morning? _____

6. Do you wake up to an alarm or naturally? _____

7. Do you feel tired in the morning or energized for the day? _____

   _____

Stress Management:

1. How is your stress level during the week day?

   _____

   _____

   _____

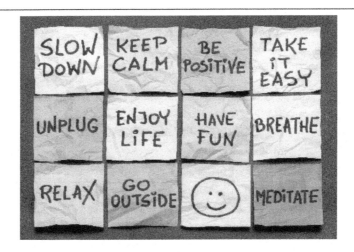

2. Do you feel irritable?
   ❏ Yes ❏ No

3. Are you an anxious person?
   ❏ Yes ❏ No

4. Do you get impatient easily?
   ❏ Yes ❏ No

5. Do you get migraines frequently or have other health issues as a result from stress?
   ❏ Yes ❏ No

6. How do you manage your stress?

   _____

   _____

   _____

   _____

7. Do you measure your heart rate variability each morning?
   ❏ Yes ❏ No

Movement:

1. How many hours do you sit during the day? Consecutive hours?

   _____

   _____

   _____

   _____

2. How much time do you spend watching television and reading electronic devices (computer, iPad, Kindle, etc.) per day?

   _____

   _____

_____

_____

3. How many steps do you take per day on average?

    _____

4. Do you use a tracking device as a Fitbit, Garmin, or Apple Watch?
    ❑ Yes   ❑ No

Digestion and Gut Health:

1. Do you feel bloated or have gas after eating any specific food?
    ❑ Yes   ❑ No
2. Do you poop at least once daily?
    ❑ Yes   ❑ No
3. Do you have any skin rash or other skin problems?
    ❑ Yes   ❑ No
4. Do you have indigestion after eating specific food?
    ❑ Yes   ❑ No

Hydration:

1. How much water do you drink per day?

    _____

    _____

    _____

2. Do you drink coffee or caffeinated beverages? How many per day?

    _____

    _____

    _____

3. Do you get headaches during the day?
   ❏ Yes   ❏ No

Happiness:

1. What makes you laugh?

   _____

   _____

   _____

   _____

2. Do you have one or more friends that you can trust and rely on each day besides your spouse?
   ❏ Yes   ❏ No

3. On Mondays, do you live for the day or live for Friday?
   ❏ Yes   ❏ No

EXERCISE #2: SPECIFIC GOAL SETTING

These are the main areas of opportunity I want to focus on to help lose fat, get healthier, and improve performance?

1. _____
2. _____
3. _____
4. _____
5. _____

I will take the following steps to reach these goals:

1. _____ Date: _____
2. _____ Date: _____

3. _____ Date: _____

4. _____ Date: _____

5. _____ Date: _____

The specific benefits I will gain by taking these steps include:

_____

_____

_____

_____

_____

I will reward myself for successfully taking these steps by:

_____

_____

_____

_____

_____

Lifestyle Habits:

To achieve my health goals, I will take the following five steps:

1. _____ Date: _____

2. _____ Date: _____

3. _____ Date: _____

4. _____ Date: _____

5. _____ Date: _____

Additional Goals (sleep, smoking, alcohol, etc.):

1. _____ Date: _____

2. _____ Date: _____

3. _____ Date: _____

4. _____ Date: _____

5. _____ Date: _____

Challenges and Solutions:

The challenges I will face in reaching my goals include:

_____

_____

_____

_____

_____

I will overcome these challenges by:

_____

_____

_____

_____

Evaluation of Goals:

Set up a reminder on your calendar to review goal. I plan to review these goals on: _____

Date: _____

Identify Your Sources of Happiness and Energy Suckers

*Lessons from Dr. Wilson in his book "Adrenal Fatigue: 21st Century Stress Syndrome.
Learn more at* https://adrenalfatigue.org/dr-wilsons-guide-to-de-stressing/

Establish what is GOOD for me and what is BAD for me

Take a piece of paper and draw a line down the middle. Make a list of "GOOD" things in your life that make you happy. Then, make a list of "BAD" things that don't make you happy.

➢ List what moves your soul. What makes you happy?

_____

_____

_____

_____

_____

➤ List what makes you unhappy? Stressed? Grumpy? Angry?

_____

_____

_____

_____

_____

1. List in order and prioritize 1-10 how many items are on your list.

    1) _____

    2) _____

    3) _____

    4) _____

    5) _____

    6) _____

    7) _____

    8) _____

    9) _____

   10) _____

2. Take the top five and then dig deeper, peel the next layer.

_____

_____

_____

_____

3. What makes those top five "GOOD" or "BAD" for your health, wellness, and mindset?

_____

_____

_____

_____

4.   Take the first item on the "BAD" list and start tackling the negative "thing" in your life for the next month. What can you change or adjust to eliminate the item or improve the situation?

_____

_____

_____

_____

5.   Make another list of health "robbers" - sources of stress or toxicity as people, workplace, family, food habits, exercise, or personal mindset. They are probably already on your "BAD" list.

_____

_____

_____

_____

6.   Take the list of "robbers" and make notes on how you can improve or change those items.

_____

_____

_____

_____

7.   After one month of focusing on improving the one "BAD" item then work on the next item on your prioritized list.

_____

_____

_____

_____

8. Also, try to work on getting more items on your "GOOD" list – what can you do to create more happiness in your life? What makes you laugh and smile? How could you do that more often?

_____

_____

_____

_____

9. Recreate your "list" in two months and reassess your happiness level and stress levels. Hopefully you made progress and on your road to a more positive healthy living environment.

STEP #2
THE WHOLESTIC METHOD ROADMAP

One of my mentors, Todd Durkin, always has our mastermind team "dig deep" to create the life we deserve. I want to "pay it forward" and help you create a roadmap to your future, so you can take action and responsibility for your health and well-being. It doesn't matter what level of athlete you are in life or if you have a specific amount of weight to lose. It only matters that you take care of yourself first.

To find out "why" and to create an action plan to help you reach your goals and dreams, we need to layout and establish the foundation. As Todd tells us: "get your mind right." We are taught in our "TD Mastermind" that to create greatness in our life, we need to discover what our passion and purpose is in our life.

Even if you are just in The WHOLESTIC Method program to drop weight, there is always a deeper meaning to why you have extra weight to lose or why you have health problems. Let's work together to establish how you can improve your life right now and then take action as we begin this transformation process and start a new journey to improve the WHOLE you.

Next, we can work on evaluating where you are in your life now. Give it a try...

EXERCISE #1: CHART YOURSELF ON THE 8 FORMS OF WEALTH

Learn more about the "8 Forms of Wealth" with Rob Sharma. Are you wealthy in life? How do you measure success in wealth? How do you get to be a world-class individual? Your mental focus and your physical energy are the most important areas to focus on in order to be world class.

Read the link (http://tinyurl.com/8FormsOfWealth) and do the exercise below.

Your inner life is what we are working on during our twenty-one-day journey together.

1. Inner life – who you are, your spiritual life, your values. How comfortable are you being you? Your self-worth. What kind of peace of mind you have. Your quality of thinking. Your inner life reflects your outer life.

2. Health life – reflects your inner life, as well. Exercise, conditioning, quality of food you eat, your sleep. We must take personal responsibility for our own health. We must be selfish in our own time to get in our workouts (as a trainer). Treat your body like the temple it is. If you don't have your health, you don't have your life.

3. Family life – Are you spending time with your family. How are your relationships with your family? When things are good at home and you're happy, you'll do better at work. Don't have regrets at the end of your life regarding your family time.

4. Career life – Are you where you want to be in your career? Are you so good that people can't take your eyes off you in your career? Did you do or are you trying to be the best in the world?

5. Economic life – Money is important, but it's not the most important. Money does make life easier and affords you a comfortable life with a nice house, nice things, and more time with the family.

6. Circle of genius – When you spend a lot of time with people, their personality, mindset, etc. rubs off on you. Always make sure you surround yourself with the best people possible.

7. Adventure success – We need to be challenged in our lives to truly be happy. We crave mystery and novelty, creativity, and joy. Meet new people. Visit new places. Eat new foods. Dare.

8. Impact life – We all want to be significant, make a difference and be part of something greater than us. We want to leave a legacy.

To Do:
1. Rate yourself on a scale from 1-10 for each of the 8 Forms of Wealth (1 being poor, 10 being "where you want to be.")

2. Plot your rating on each of the axis in the circle that corresponds to each of the 8 Forms of Wealth.

3. Connect the dots. This makes a nice visual of where you might want to focus some of your efforts. Ideally, you want a circle as big as the one below.

Todd Durkin always tells us in our mastermind group: "*A leader of one, a leader of many. If you can't lead one, you can't lead any."* This is so true.

Now, stop and think about one or two action steps you can do to elevate your career right now.

1. Do you listen to podcasts or TED Talks?

   ❑ Yes   ❑ No

   If so, which are your favorites? _____

   _____

   _____

   _____

   _____

2. How do you keep up with news and research?

   _____

   _____

   _____

   _____

   _____

3. How do you challenge your brain?

   _____

   _____

   _____

   _____

   _____

4. Do you surround yourself with people who are "smarter" than you?

❏ Yes   ❏ No

Explain:

_____

_____

_____

_____

5. Do you take action on a project, but are afraid of the risk and your ability to follow through to the end result?

❏ Yes   ❏ No

Explain:

_____

_____

_____

_____

Financial wealth – Time freedom and money freedom. What financial number would you like to achieve by end of the year? Money buys freedom. What can you do to boost your salary? What can you do to improve your status? Are you involved in supporting your church or other organization financially? Who are you going to give your money to in life?

Dash-mark - To be the best in the world, you must be one percent (1%) better every day. The impact is created because of the intention you have to do better.

Let's create awareness of where we are in these life areas to become world class. As we increase our awareness in these areas, we can make better choices which lead to better results.

Next, rank yourself on a scale of 1-10. 1 = poor and 10 = world class in each of these eight forms of wealth.

Where do you rank the highest? Where am I lowest?

Those are your areas of opportunities. We want to measure where we need to spend time focusing in order to be more world class and successful from the inside out.

Then, create a graph via the chart provided to make a bar graph.

Next, we will work on setting three goals for each area we need to focus on to complete in thirty days.

Here you go... in the next thirty days, you will:

1. _____
2. _____
3. _____
4. _____
5. _____

To read and learn more about "8 Forms of Wealth" exercise:
http://www.robinsharma.com/resources
http://tinyurl.com/UndergroundWellnessPodcast

EXERCISE #2: REFLECTION

Take time for gratitude. Reflect on the past year and look forward to the next one.

1. Who are you most grateful for in your life?

_____
_____
_____
_____
_____

2. What are you most grateful in your life?

_____

_____

_____

_____

_____

3.   What do you want to accomplish in the upcoming year?
   a.   Personal: _____
   b.   Business: _____
   c.   Spiritual: _____
   d.   Physical: _____
   e.   Health: _____

4.   What are your best habits and practices you find that provide you success in all areas of life?
   a.   Personal: _____
   b.   Business: _____
   c.   Spiritual: _____
   d.   Physical: _____
   e.   Health: _____

5.   What are the areas of opportunity for you to improve upon this year to be the best you?
   a.   Personal: _____
   b.   Business: _____
   c.   Spiritual: _____
   d.   Physical: _____
   e.   Health: _____

6.   What is one major area that you need to focus on improving this year?
   a.   Personal: _____
   b.   Business: _____
   c.   Spiritual: _____
   d.   Physical: _____
   e.   Health: _____

7.   Create a vision board... where do you see yourself in five years and ten years?

    a.   Personal: _____

    b.   Business: _____

    c.   Spiritual: _____

    d.   Physical: _____

    e.   Health: _____

8.   What is a struggle for you now that you need to focus on creating strategies to overcome?

_____

_____

_____

_____

9.   Which WHOLESTIC Method element do you think you should focus on right now for the next thirty days?

_____

_____

_____

_____

_____

10. What is moving or driving you right now to change yourself from the inside out?

_____

_____

_____

_____

_____

11. What do you need to not focus on so much? Where are you losing time, or wasting energy?

_____

_____

_____

_____

_____

_____

12. What are your action steps to create an area of opportunity to grow from the inside out in the next two to four months?

_____

_____

_____

_____

_____

_____

13. What is your purpose in life? I always believe everything happens for a reason and we discover through experiences which road our journey is taking us on. Where is your road taking you?

_____

_____

_____

_____

_____

_____

14. What makes you smile, laugh, and be happy?

_____

_____

_____

_____

_____

15. What makes you motivated and drives you to wake up each day?

_____

_____

_____

_____
_____
_____

16. On the flip side, what makes you anxious, nervous, or stressed out?

_____
_____
_____
_____
_____
_____
_____

17. What scares you the most that may be a roadblock to taking care of yourself?

_____
_____
_____
_____
_____
_____

18. What or who makes your angry and/or frustrated?

_____
_____
_____
_____
_____

19. What or who makes you run away and avoid a situation or an experience?

_____
_____
_____
_____

_____
_____

20. What is your "WHY" to improve your fat loss, health, or performance?

_____
_____
_____
_____
_____

21. Are you motivated to make those daily lifestyle changes to be the best version of yourself?

   ❑ Yes❑ No

22. Would you want to live anywhere other than where you live now?

   ❑ Yes❑ No

23. Do you love your home? Workplace? Do these places make you smile?

   ❑ Yes❑ No

   ❑ Yes❑ No

   ❑ Yes❑ No

24. Do you relax at home and enjoy spending time alone, or would you rather be with a group of people? Explain.

_____
_____
_____
_____
_____
_____

25. How many vacations do you take per year?

_____

26. How often are you on your phone and checking/reading emails each day?

_____

27. Do you set time limits or schedule when you are available via phone, text, or email?
❑ Yes ❑ No

28. Do you disconnect from your computer, emails, and social media on vacations or weekends?
❑ Yes ❑ No

29. What time do you go to bed ideally? What time do you wake up naturally?

_____

_____

30. How would your spouse describe you? Your best friend? Your parents?

_____

_____

_____

_____

31. How many hours do you work per day? Per week?

_____

32. Do you have any fears?
❑ Yes ❑ No

33. What are your dreams? Big wish list?

_____

_____

_____

_____

_____

34. Do you have a strong relationship with your spouse or partner?
❑ Yes ❑ No

35. What causes you the most stress each day?

_____
_____
_____
_____
_____
_____

36. What could you do to improve to begin the day happy and energetic?

_____
_____
_____
_____
_____
_____

37. How could you improve your sleep? What evening rituals would help you relax and unwind?

_____
_____
_____
_____
_____
_____

38. Do you feel you look and feel your best from the inside out?
❏ Yes❏ No
If not, how could you improve your opinion of yourself? _____

_____
_____
_____
_____

Do you have a habit you want to change that annoys you, but you don't know how to break and/or create a permanent change?
❏ Yes❏ No

Explain: _____
_____

_____

_____

_____

_____

EXERCISE #3: THE EIGHT ELEMENTS OF THE WHOLESTIC METHOD

Let's see where you are in the eight elements of The WHOLESTIC Method, which are all important areas to improve in order to reach our goals, as a lack in one area impact another area. For example, if you are stressed out each day, then your sleep will be impacted, you make poor food choices, and your workouts lack focus and effort. Stress can then impact gut health as the gut and brain are connected. You get the picture.

Review your current area for opportunity of the eight elements of The WHOLESTIC Method to transform the WHOLE you. Where are you right now on a scale one (worst case) to ten (ideal) in each element?

Here we go:

1. NUTRITION:____
2. EXERCISE:____
3. SLEEP:____
4. STRESS:____
5. MOVEMENT:____
6. GUT HEALTH/DIGESTION:____
7. HYDRATION:____
8. HAPPINESS:____

EXERCISE #4: GET YOUR LIFE ORGANIZED

My mentors, Todd Durkin (http://todddurkin.com) and Larry Indiviglia, have our mastermind group complete Wayne Cotton's color-coded calendar each year and create our own annual roadmap. You can create your own roadmap toward transforming the WHOLE you with the tools provided in The WHOLESTIC Method manual.

Focus on how you can make more time for taking self-care, as with your nutrition, exercise, sleep, stress, movement, digestion/gut health, hydration, and happiness.

1. Fill out a color-coded calendar (Annual Roadmap) from Wayne Cotton. Download a sample roadmap and a blank one at http://nobrowndays.com/

2. Fill out a calendar with four different colors (yellow, blue, red, and green) so your entire year is color-coded. Start with "mellow yellow," build in "blue-sky" days two to three days per quarter, and then fill in "green machine" and "red tape."

3. Take a picture of you today and then visualize how you want to see yourself from the inside out one year from now. Write on the back of the photo or in a journal how you feel now and how you think of yourself when you look at your photo. Would you want to change any of your thoughts on how you look and feel from the inside out?

Let's review a method that helps create more time in each area of your life. See how you can schedule more "blue sky" and "yellow mellow" time if that is what is needed. Maybe you need to schedule in "red tape" time if you are like me and dislike financials or accounting, but it is something you must do. Above you identified what moves your soul… and what robs you of energy. Now, prioritize what you can do to make more time for creating happiness in your life as all the other The WHOLESTIC Method elements will improve if you are feeling happy and energized about life. (Homework: Inspired by one of mentors Todd Durkin)

Color code your life:

Color coding your life to improve the WHOLE you from the inside out is a system created by Wayne Cotton and recommended by my business coach, Todd Durkin. Please visit www.nobrowndays.com for free information on learning about the definition of each color, as well as check a video (http://tinyurl.com/ColorCodingLife) with Todd Durkin and Wayne Cotton detailing the system.

What does each color mean to you/your inner life?

a.   Green Machine: _____

b.   Blue Sky Time: _____

c.Red Tape Time: _____

d.   Mellow Yellow Time: _____

Complete a Ninety Day Wonder every three months.

a.   What have I accomplished in the last ninety days?

_____

_____

_____

_____

b.   What are my current challenges?

_____

_____

_____

_____

c.What will I accomplish in the next ninety days?

_____

_____

_____

_____

Pick five big projects you want to complete monthly.

a.   This month you want to work on which projects?

1. _____

2. _____

3. _____

4. _____

5. _____

b.   List how you are going to specifically complete them each project... set five mini sub goals for each item.

1. _____

2. _____

3. _____

4. _____

5. _____

c. Who can you be accountable to take and be successful in completing these life changing personal projects?

1. _____

2. _____

3. _____

4. _____

5. _____

Every week, pick five projects you want to complete in the week to help get you to your thirty-day goals. Write them down Sunday evening in your weekly calendar.

Every day, pick five things you want to tackle and complete to help get you to your weekly goals. Write them down on your daily calendar and check them off when completed.

Inspiration from my mentor: Todd Durkin http://www.todddurkin.com/

EXERCISE #5: WHAT IS YOUR "DASH?"

When we pass away, we leave a legacy. The author of the poem, *The Dash*, Linda Ellis, writes an amazing verse that opens your eyes to what you do with your life. She says our tombstone will have two dates on it: the one when we were born and the one when we pass away. However, in between the dates is a dash. The dash represents your entire life. (Visit the link below to read the entire copyrighted poem.)

What do you want to do with your life? I am sure you don't want to feel rushed every day, racing through the day being distracted and unfocused. Nor do you wish to be on a diet trying to lose weight every few months. We often live each day looking ahead and not living in the present.

What if today was your last? What would you regret not doing? Who do you wish you would have spent more time with before you pass away? Where do you want to travel to or visit? If tomorrow was your last day alive, would you be happy about who you are today and the life you've lived? If not, what would you change? Maybe you wish you had a more positive outlook on life? Or that you'd slowed down to enjoy your coffee outside in the backyard and watched the birds and squirrels play in the trees?

I have discovered from my own experiences that most of us spend way too much time concerned about other people (worry), what's happening on our cell phones (addiction), what are we missing out on (fear), as well as what other people think of themselves and not enough time focusing on how we feel about ourselves. Are you fulfilled in your life so far today? What does your intuition say about you? Listen to your gut and start working from the inside out to learn about how you want to live your "dash."

Now, it is time to write your legacy. Take at least fifteen minutes in a quiet and relaxing space to write out how you visualize your celebration of life, as well as what people would say about you. Then, write your obituary.

How is your eulogy going to read?

http://www.linda-ellis.com/the-dash-the-dash-poem-by-linda-ellis-.html

Write your own "dash." _____

_____

_____

_____

_____

_____

_____

_____

_____

STEP #3
WORKING FROM THE INSIDE OUT TO TRANSFORM THE WHOLE YOU

How can you get started right now on becoming a fat burner instead of a sugar burner? We need to discuss each of the eight elements of The WHOLESTIC Method before we start your new journey. Get ready to read the manual and then get a pen out for the workbook as you will be creating your roadmap to transforming the WHOLE you from the inside out.

Let's start by answering the questions in the Roadmap Workbook to help you "work in" before we "work out." Then, we'll determine what you need to focus on first:

Get a Team: Recruit a team to join the journey with you. Communicate your goals to your family and friends. Support is needed from people at home, work, and social events. Check out our Facebook Group pages and www.thewholesticmethod.com coaching program.

Accountability: Connect daily with your team and coach as much as possible. Share your challenge with your family, friends, and co-workers to help keep you accountable and honest.

Measure, Monitor, and Track your Exercise:

- Use MYZONE heart rate training to track exercise. Learn how to order and set up your MYZONE heart rate belt and use our facility code to join our team... FITFORUS001
- Set up and use your belt using these instructions: http://tinyurl.com/MYZONETraining
- Download the SweetBeat Life app to monitor your daily stress, recovery, and more with the MYZONE heart rate monitor. http://tinyurl.com/SweetbeatFeatures

Communication: For best results, connect with your coach and teammates each day to ask for help and support when struggling.

Motivate: Support. Inspire. Impact. EVERYDAY.

Journal: Keep a log of when you eat, why you eat, and where you are eating to learn about your eating habits. Track your sleep, mood, and stress levels. Journal any stressful experiences, struggles, and obstacles and then list solutions to overcome the roadblocks.

Focus: To get the results you are looking for, communicate, plan ahead, be prepared, and be organized. Set weekly goals every Sunday and daily goals—your big five for the week and each day—and review them nightly to keep your mind right.

Positive Attitude: Get your mindset right. We are creating new lifestyle habits, so be mentally prepared. Keeping a gratitude journal will help you see the positive changes. Have the attitude of gratitude. We will learn how to enjoy being in the present and seeing each day as a gift instead of living in the past or the future. Be in the moment and focus on the good in your life.

Collect Baseline Data: Take your photo, bodyweight, and measurements day one and at end of the 21-plus days. Continue to weigh in once a week and take measurements once a month after doing the program to keep on track. You don't know how far you have improved if you don't know where you started.

Lab Testing: See the detailed lab testing links on http://thewholesticmethod.com.

Be Organized: Plan your meals weekly. Included in your manual is a copy of my Phase One program I provide to my coaching clients. The 5-Day Jumpstart Challenge offers a sample meal plan as well as food you can eat lists for our jumpstart Sugar Detox and Reset program to get started on The WHOLESTIC Method approach to fat loss, health, and performance.

Print out your shopping lists and make copies of your daily food log. Also, suggested cookbooks are included as the Ketogenic Cookbooks by Maria Emmerich, Primal Blueprint Easy and Quick Meals on www.marksdailyapple.com and The Practical Paleo cookbook by Diane Sanfilippo.

Finally, see our Pinterest Pages including Low-Carb High-Fat meals and much more on my The WHOLESTIC Method boards.

Grocery Shop and Cook Extras Weekly: Go grocery shopping every few days since you are buying fresh and local organic vegetables whenever possible. Sundays are a great day to get prepared and organized, plus even make extra meals for leftovers to take to work for lunch.

Schedule Your Personal Time: Look ahead and block out your time including relaxation time and workouts. Schedule your workouts into your daily schedule. Try to spend ten minutes every Sunday to set up your Weekly Exercise Structure plan for the week ahead and block out time on your calendar - sacred time.

Prioritize You: Remember to pack workout clothes and shoes each day. Make appointments with yourself to MOVE every thirty minutes. Plan your weekly workouts. Register for your personal training sessions on our FITNESS FORWARD STUDIO registration link at www.mindbodyonline.com, so you receive reminders or at your own studio.

That's it.

It's that simple.

Now, once you have read about the eight elements of The WHOLESTIC Method in the manual section, we are ready to tackle The WHOLESTIC Method Workbook section to get started on your new journey to improve the WHOLE you from the inside out.

HOW TO IMPROVE THE WHOLE YOU:

1. Determine what are your obstacles and challenges to being successful in the next five days?

2. What are your solutions to overcoming those challenges?
   a. How are you going to create those challenges into opportunities to improve and grow?
   b. Celebrate what you do have now and find the joy in this new journey in becoming the new and improved version of yourself.
   c. The 5-Day challenge is not just crossing the finish line in five days, but starting a new journey that continues. Be present and enjoy the process not always focusing on the outcome.

3. Visualize. In order to create new habits and lifestyle changes, we need to make some adjustments:
   - You can do more of some things
   - You can do less of other things
   - You can start doing something you have not done before
   - You can stop doing something that is not helpful in achieving your goals.

Incorporate each trick below for five days; you will make a shift in your health, life, and performance to improve the WHOLE you from the inside out.

1. **Nutrition**: Eat REAL FOOD based on your biochemical individuality. In Phase One, we are giving our digestion system a break and detoxing our liver pathways; Phase Two

will introduce more food, yet still eliminating common food sensitivities and inflammatory foods.

- Eat one nutritious shake per day (directions below)
- One or more fresh, super green drink per day (no fruit added)
- One big meal per day with vegetables, protein, and healthy fat – ideally mid-afternoon and a light snack or shake in evenings.
- Eat lots of vegetables, healthy fats, and lean proteins for main meal: organic and free-range source protein when possible.
- Eliminate inflammatory foods such as gluten, grains, processed foods, manufactured/factory-made foods, GMO soy, corn, and peanuts. Cut out commercial dairy to test sensitivity (raw sheep or goat cheese is often better on gut and digestion)
- Try adding "Amazing Grass Greens" or another source of greens to your water each day.
- Remember to stop eating two hours before bed and eat your main meal in the afternoon (ideally). Kitchen closed. Drink water.
- You should feel energized and satisfied, not starving.

2. **Exercise:**
   - Add three sessions per week of thirty-minute total body strength training workouts with cardio blasts to spike post workout metabolism (green/yellow-red zones if wearing MyZone heart rate monitor)
   - Three sessions of thirty minutes or more walking, biking, hiking, running... (blue/green zone)
   - Wear MYZONE for all exercise sessions to earn MYZONE Effort Points (MEPs)
   - Schedule shared personal training thirty-minute sessions or group training sessions

3. **Sleep:**
   - Get to bed by 10:00 p.m. or earlier to get your seven to nine hours per night.
   - Wind down before bed: read in bed, dim the lights, and empty your mind (journals help... see section on Happiness)
   - Listen to my podcast for sleep ideas, as well as the chapter on sleep in The WHOLESTIC Method manual.

- Test your daily heart rate variability using the MYZONE heart rate monitor and the SweetBeat Life app on your iPhone for three to five minutes every morning.

4. **Stress:**
   - Determine triggers and solutions to improve stress – the first part of the workbook should help you identify your energy robbers.
   - Measure heart rate variability each morning three to five minutes (download the SweetBeat Life app on your phone and use your MyZone Bluetooth monitor)
   - Detox relationships by improving or changing toxic people in your life (make sure to do an inner-work section in the workbook before you start Phase One.)
   - Slow down and give more time in between appointments or day. Block out time for you each day on your schedule and prioritize time for you each day

5. **Movement:**
   - Track movement – 10,000 steps per day with tracking device of your choice.
   - Get up and move every hour
   - Make a note on your desk or set the timer to get up and walk around, squat, lunge, twist and rotate if sitting most of the day... move.

6. **Digestion, Gut & Hormone Health:**
   - Eat naturally fermented foods like sauerkraut, cultured vegetables, natural apple cider vinegar and foods rich in probiotics (kefir)
   - Take a probiotic each morning (see website for suggestions and links
   - Add fermented foods into diet – as kraut juice into green drinks
   - Fish oil with vitamin D each day
   - You may benefit from taking digestive enzyme and HCL with your meal each day if signs or history of acid reflux or GERD.
   - Gut healing will occur over time when you eliminate gluten, processed foods, inflammatory foods (as excessive Omega 6-vegetable oils) and sugar
   - Get lab testing (see WellnessFX link on web page or resources) to determine supplement need, thyroid health, gut biome, hormones, and more.

7. **Hydration:**
   - Drink half your body weight of water in ounces throughout day

- Add Himalayan sea salt and lemon
- Drink the detox water drink each day with apple cider vinegar (1-2 tablespoons) plus lemon and cayenne pepper (some people add cinnamon as well.)
- No alcohol during the program - phase one especially.
- Limit coffee (organic source) to two cups per day; only before 12:00 p.m.

8. **Happiness:**
   - Laugh aloud each day
   - Listen to music in your car or home that you love but also calms and relaxes you
   - Surround yourself with people who make you smile and laugh
   - Do one thing each day that brings you joy, smiles, and laughter
   - Go play on the weekends with family or friends or simply unplug
   - Massage, foot reflexology or spa day

THE PRE-5-DAY JUMPSTART CHALLENGE REMINDERS:

Be sure to read **The WHOLESTIC Method 5-Day Jumpstart Challenge** manual plus the paperwork on the new client forms link on my website: www.debbiepotts.net. You'll receive the 5-Day manual after you register online for the program.

Secret Detox Drink - Dr. Axe:

https://draxe.com/recipe/secret-detox-drink

Ingredients:

1 glass of warm or hot water (12-16 ounces)

2 tablespoons apple cider vinegar

2 tablespoons lemon juice

½-1 teaspoon ground ginger

¼ teaspoon cinnamon

1 dash cayenne pepper

I suggest adding this daily supplement drink for thirty days or more to help balance blood sugar, brain health, and ability to focus:

https://thewholesticmethod.pruvitnow.com/product/ketoos-2-1-orange-dream

You can learn more about ketones via this link. Watch this short five-minute video:

https://www.youtube.com/watch?v=mpl2om711cM

PRE-5-DAY JUMPSTART CHALLENGE PREPARATION:

- No eating after 8:00 p.m., so finish your meal or shake before then.
- Send in accountability report to my Facebook page or website www.thewholesticmethod.com.
- Check out my cooking and exercise videos on my YouTube channel (http://tinyurl.com/FitForYouTube) if you need ideas and workouts. Subscribe so you can get updates.
- Share food pictures of your main daily meal on our Facebook group page. I shared a photo of my simple and quick meal I made: Turkey, broccoli, cauliflower, kale, and Brussels sprout slaw.
- Complete the metabolic type form and health appraisal form for your information. Then, highlight the areas you scored on (health form) to focus on improving or figuring out your "Why?"
- Here are the forms and Amazon links http://tinyurl.com/FitForAmzLinks.
- A daily accountability email will be sent for the next five days to keep you on the program and following the guidelines.
- Keep it simple: NSNG = NO SUGAR and NO GRAINS.
- Included in your daily accountability report will be...
- Homework - read http://tinyurl.com/FatLossInfluencer

Here are the basics to the Phase One: 5-Day Jumpstart Challenge:

1. Drink vegetable juice, detox water, tea, and water with sea salt.
2. Eat one big meal per day in the late afternoon or early evening = higher healthy fats, moderate protein, and low carbohydrate (vegetables).
3. Low-carb, high-fat real food plan, but eat when hungry not by the time of day.
4. Snack if hungry. See food list for ideas (low carb ideas that will fill you up and keep you full longer)
5. One shake (or two if more active) with water or add a healthy fat to keep more satiated as coconut milk or nut butter for more of a meal replacement
6. Add one or two packets per day of Prüvit Keto/OS into your water for brain power and exogenous ketones (see more in nutrition chapter about ketones). Buy at http://thewholesticmethod.pruvitnow.com/.
7. Apply other The WHOLESTIC Method guidelines in the manual for nutrition, exercise, sleep, stress, digestion, hydration, movement, and happiness.
8. Keep a journal throughout the program including your gratitude for each day.

I dislike the word "diet," so I refer to The WHOLESTIC Method's food direction as a short-term eating plan. If we could learn how to eat right for our metabolic type and to do it only when we are hungry instead of mindless snacking around the clock, then how much more energy may surprise us we have as well as noticeable health improvements.

Our secret to fat loss is to eat REAL FOOD and then take care of your other elements. See the forms on my web page to get started on the health appraisal and metabolic type questionnaire: www.thewholesticmethod.com.

1. Take this METABOLIC TYPE test (www.thewholesticmethod.com) if you really want to know what ratio of macronutrients (fat/protein/carb) for your metabolic type. Are you a protein/fat type, mixed or carb type?
2. Clean out the pantry and fridge. Take a picture and send it to me via our program website www.thewholesticmethod.com. Remove bread, pasta, crackers, cookies, chips, and all other refined sugar processed foods. Don't throw anything away, but instead donate it to a food shelter, charity, or church pantry.
3. Make a shopping list and head to your local quality grocery store. Stock up for the week and restock your fridge with local and organic fresh foods. Healthy fats, grass-fed meat, wild fish, local organic vegetables, and some local berries.

4. Send pictures of your pantry, fridge, and meals to your coach as well as to our private Facebook page:

5. Costco (or similar warehouse store) shopping list:
   - ☐ Avocados
   - ☐ Organic spinach, kale, and other vegetables
   - ☐ Organic Coconut Oil
   - ☐ Extra Virgin Olive Oil and/or avocado oil
   - ☐ Organic Chia Seeds
   - ☐ Saigon Cinnamon - organic
   - ☐ Kerry Gold butter or other pasture butter
   - ☐ Raw walnuts and almonds
   - ☐ Free range meat and poultry
   - ☐ Wild salmon or other seafood
   - ☐ Free range organic eggs

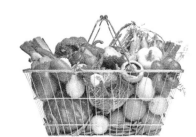

6. Shop at the local Farmers Market when possible

7. Proteins: grass-fed or wild caught. Land, sea, or air.

8. Fats: Coconut oil, EVOO, avocado, macadamia, olives, fresh cream, sardines, walnuts, and almonds.

9. Vegetables: colorful, local, organic, in season, ideally.

10. Fruit: Limit fruit intake if fat loss the goal, except for berries.

11. Avoid: grains gluten, sugar, corn, soy, commercial dairy, peanuts, and processed foods. Less than five (understandable) ingredients on the label.

What Should We Eat: Primal Nutrition - Real Food?

Don't focus on what you can't have but all the amazing foods you can eat and enjoy and taste. Organic and local foods have much more flavor and taste.

We should eat anything that is grown, hunted, or picked.

Avoid processed, packaged foods, sugars, genetically-modified foods, as well as common food allergens or inflammatory foods like gluten/grains, commercial dairy, soy, and peanuts.

- Select any type of organic, healthy, free-range, pasture proteins.
- Select any of healthy fats listed on our food list.
- Eat many colorful organic, fresh, in-season, local vegetables.

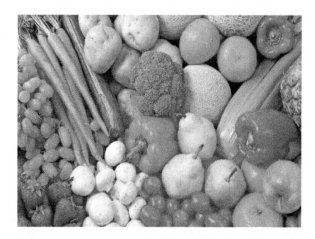

Carbohydrates:

- Eat lots of organic, colorful vegetables at all meals
- Limit fruits for the 21 to 30-day challenge (or add organic berries)
- Low glycemic and non-starchy vegetables (high fiber)
- Avoid gluten and grains, including processed gluten-free products
- Avoid sugar and high fructose corn syrup
- Try limiting carbohydrates to 50-100 grams per day on non-workout days and 100-150 grams on longer workout days if trying to go low-carb for 21 days.

Protein:

- Protein should be grass-fed, wild, free range, and organic
- If needed, use Pea (vegan) or Whey Protein powder (organic, farm-raised whey protein, least amount of processing) for shakes
- Fish (wild, not farm raised)
- Free roaming (cage free), organic, local eggs
- Full fat plain Greek yogurt (limit commercial dairy or eliminate for month)
- Tempeh (limit soy, especially GMO)

Fats:

- Organic wild fish and fish oils
- Fresh organic and raw nut butter (fat/protein/carbs) – not roasted in vegetable oils and added sugar (read ingredients).
- Organic Olive and Coconut Oils (cook with olive oil only at low heat)
- Avocados, olives, sardines

- Raw nuts and seeds (unsalted and not roasted)
- Real coconut milk, cream, flakes, and oil – unsweetened (read ingredients)
- Raw goat or sheep cheeses (avoid cow), if doing dairy
- Full organic yogurt and fat heavy cream, if doing dairy
- Grass-fed butter (organic grass fed and free range)

One Big Meal per Day: ideally, eat this meal at mid-afternoon or ask me if intermittent fasting is appropriate for you (more later in the manual.)

Suggested Supplements: Get lab testing from WellnessFX (see www.thewholesticmethod.com for lab testing), but here are possible supplements to your diet:

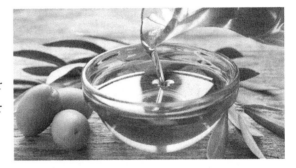

- Omega 3 - Fish Oil or Cod Liver Oil
- Probiotics
- Vitamin D 3
- BCAA: especially if exercising higher intensities and/or longer duration or vegan
- Vitamin C
- Vitamin B12
- Magnesium (Epsom Gel if muscle pain or great before bed to help sleep)
- Cinnamon – helps blood sugar balance and metabolism
- Maca Powder - http://macapowderbenefits.net/
- Glutamine 500-1000 mg if sugar cravings or gut damage

Additional Notes:
- Take .5-.70-gram protein x bodyweight = _____ protein per day (amount depends on individual)
- Distribute protein and fat at each meal with vegetables.

Drink half your body weight in ounces of water per day: _____body weight/2 = _____ ounces per day

STEP #4
PHASE ONE:
THE WHOLESTIC METHOD
5-DAY DETOX & RESET
JUMPSTART CHALLENGE

Our lifestyle and eating habits are a choice we make every day. Today, you have decided to take control and ownership of your health. If we want to feel better, look better, and move better, then we need to make smarter decisions by working on the WHOLE individual from the inside out. Instead of cutting calories and exercising more to lose weight, we are going to re-train the brain when we need to eat, why we are eating, and what we need to eat to feel satisfied and happy.

Do you want to feel happy, energetic, and sleep well every day?

Yes.

Let's stop self-sabotaging ourselves and figure out our "Why" by improving our health from the inside out with my WHOLESTIC Method. We are going to work on the WHOLE you with my 5-Day Jumpstart Detox & Reset Challenge (Phase One), then you can choose if you would like to continue improving the WHOLE you with my twenty-one day WHOLESTIC Method coaching program (Phase Two).

The WHOLESTIC Method covers eight elements to improve fat loss, health, and performance:

The 5-day challenge is a jumpstart on a sugar detox and reset challenge with The WHOLESTIC Method approach to work on the WHOLE you from the inside out. We are getting serious in the first five days, then you can continue for twenty-one or more days committing on these new WHOLESTIC habits to create lasting change.

The WHOLESTIC Method 5-Day Jumpstart Challenge is designed to help introduce new eating habits to you, as well as learning about our relationship to food, sugar, and alcohol. The challenge will help lead you to a new world of optimal living and able to reach peak performance in life and sports. Each day, we will touch on the eight elements of The WHOLESTIC Method and set daily goals: nutrition, exercise, sleep, stress, movement, digestion/gut health, hydration, and happiness.

The 5-Day challenge is focused on eating real food and moving your body more. The WHOLESTIC Method twenty-one-day challenge will dig deeper into the eight elements of improving fat loss, health, and performance. Now, we go into eating one nutritional shake, one green vegetable drink, and one big meal per day filled with vegetables, healthy fat, and quality protein. We are going to become fat burning machines by eating more healthy fats that will burn more fat. This is completely opposite from what we have been taught our whole lives. Excess sugar and empty calorie carbohydrates are actually causing us to gain fat weight -plus leads to multiple other health issues and inflammation because of the blood sugar roller coaster we continue to ride on and create chaos with our fat storing hormones. Aren't you ready to get off the ride?

Over the next five-plus days, you will commit to each element of the program as it is laid out and you will be on your road to becoming a fat burning machine. As I said, the first five days are a jumpstart into creating changes with our eating habits, but if you continue to eat low carb and higher fat food, then you can change your body from being a sugar burner into a fat burner in two to three weeks. To become a fat burner, you need to stop being a sugar burner. How? Eat more healthy fats and lower your carbohydrates.

First, we need to find out your "Why" if we are going to work on the WHOLE you with The WHOLESTIC Method to improve fat loss, health, and performance. Then, you will be able to commit and create long-lasting change that brings success to all areas of your life from the inside out. Let's bring on the long-lasting transformation process with the 5-Day Jumpstart Challenge. Get your mind right and let's get going.

Download a free e-book to learn the eight secrets to avoiding adrenal fatigue at www.thewholesticmethod.com.

Let's get started by applying the key principles of The WHOLESTIC Method's eight elements.

1. Start by taking the Metabolic Type test – see my website link on www.thewholesticmethod.com for the health appraisal form.
2. Tell me what drives you to follow The WHOLESTIC Method program and start the detox and reset program.
3. Visit http://fitnessforwardstudio.com/home/new-clients/

Should you do a detox challenge?

We are often told to do a "detox" after the holiday season to lose weight and to feel better. I offer a The WHOLESTIC Method 5-Day Jumpstart Challenge every month for clients as well as a 21-day version that includes drinking a detox tea and other supplements to support the liver as well as our digestion system.

Does a detox work?

The liver has many roles in the body to keep us healthy and alive. So, when we overwhelm our liver by drinking too much alcohol, eating too much sugar or processed foods, breathing in toxic air at work, outdoors pollutants and home toxins, we need to "cleanse" the liver to keep it strong and capable of keeping up with its many roles.

As Dr. Axe said in one of his many liver cleansing articles…

"One of the main ways that the body rids itself of toxins is through the liver. In fact, the liver is one of the hardest (and largest) organs in the body. It works tirelessly to detoxify our blood, produce the bile needed to digest fat, breakdown hormones, and store essential vitamins, minerals, and irons."

Source: www.draxe.com

The liver oversees processing all the toxins entering the body, so we need the liver to be in prime condition to keep up with its job. A quarterly liver type of detox is beneficial as well as drinking "detox" teas regularly as an herbal tea with dandelion.

Research articles show the benefits of a liver detox include:

- Improved digestion of fat -since the liver produces bile that is stored in the gallbladder that is needed to emulsify fats.
- Improved immune system since the liver reduces toxins in the body then we can assume our immune system is stronger. Our immune system is our "army" to fight environmental toxins, bad bacteria, viruses, and other types of harmful microorganisms.
- Improved liver function will improve the gallbladder's bile flow which will help to avoid bile stones that form when stagnant bile because hardened and then forms little stones that can block the bile duct. When we have proper liver, gallbladder, pancreas, and small intestine, then we will have proper fat digestion, and the gallbladder will be able to release the necessary bile.
- Low-fat and non-fat diets, as well as bad-fat diets, do not trigger the release of bile, so it becomes more viscous or old leading to the gallbladder not being able to contract and release the bile, then we don't properly absorb fats that are crucial to every cell in our body.

- Improved energy and vitality since a healthy functioning liver will help us properly absorb the nutrients our body needs. If our liver has too much toxic build up, some of the nutrients may not continue into our bloodstream for uptake by the cells.

Learn more on our recent podcast, you can find on iTunes or at:

www.thewholeathletepodcast.com

Resources:

www.globalhealingcenter.com

www.draxe.com

THE 5-DAY JUMPSTART CHALLENGE DETOX SIDE EFFECTS:

No need to worry, you won't be running to the bathroom having an "explosion" each day, but you will be cleaning out your internal "filter" as you get an "oil and lube job" for your "car." Your liver and digestive systems need to be rested, restored, and recharged, as you do for your car, to function properly and to decrease the risk for health problems and diseases in our future.

During the 5-Day Jumpstart Challenge program, you may be experiencing some withdrawals from sugar, wheat, alcohol, and even caffeine. Some clients note experiencing fatigue, brain fog, skin acne, gas, mood swings, irritability, headaches, diarrhea, or constipation. Not to worry, though, most clients only experience the side effects for a few days as their body adapts to the change of eating habits. Sometimes, we are not aware of the amount of sugar, processed foods, chemicals, and alcohol in our daily diet until we remove them all. Even healthy natural sugar sources will cause blood sugar imbalance and activate the fat storing hormone insulin. The increased amount of vegetables may cause a change in the body's digestion systems, but your body will adjust, and the symptoms typically subside in a few days.

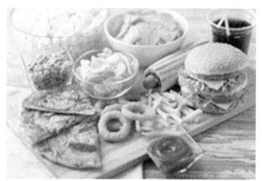

If you feel tired and fatigued, you may be not eating enough, so make sure you take the "Metabolic Type" questionnaire, so you are eating for your type and then make sure you are never starving. You should feel full and satisfied after eating a meal for three-plus hours. Try testing your blood sugar two hours after your meal. I don't want you to feel "hangry" (hungry and angry). Rather, you should be full of energy as we break the sugar addiction and improve the detox pathways.

THE 5-DAY JUMPSTART CHALLENGE MEAL PLAN THEME

- Low carb, moderate protein, and high healthy fat
- Main meal should be filled with organic vegetables, healthy fats, and quality free range/wild sources protein.
- Eliminate processed foods, sugars, commercial dairy, soy, corn, wheat/gluten, and grains. No alcohols during the 5-Day detox and reset challenge.

The 5-Day Meal Plan:
- Nutritional shake with greens and probiotics
- Main meal in afternoon: mostly organic vegetables, lean protein, and healthy fats
- Super greens drink - see recipes below
- Coffee in the morning with healthy fats – try making French Press coffee and add a tablespoon of coconut oil or MCT oil plus grass-fed butter (Kerry Gold) or in herbal tea for "Fat Coffee" then put in blender.
- Snacks if needed: cut up vegetables with olive oil or other ideas below

Beverages:

- Drink filtered water throughout the day (half your body weight in ounces of water)
- Add Himalayan sea salt to water
- Drink liver detox tea (see shopping links on www.thewholesticmethod.com)
- Detox drink - water, 1-2 tablespoons apple cider vinegar, dash of cayenne pepper, and a squeeze of lemon
- No alcohol, soda, sugar water, or processed beverages

Eating Tip: No dieting or starving

- Eat when you're hungry - if eating right macronutrient ratio and biochemical individuality (do you metabolic typing questionnaire) to find how much fats-protein-carbohydrate your body type needs based on your ancestral background.
- You should be full and satisfied for three hours or more, or else, you probably need more healthy fats in meals.
- Half your body weight in ounces of water per day with sea salt
- Prepare your nutritional shake in the morning once hungry
- Eat one meal per day, preferably in the afternoon
- Choose one meal or snacks from list below

Key Points on what to eat... keep it simple

- Everyone is different. Review your results from the Metabolic Type and Lifestyle questionnaire (download www.fitnessforwardstudio.com/fuel)
- EAT REAL WHOLE FOODS which are foods that have been picked, fished, or hunted.
- The program is based on whole, natural foods your body can fully utilize.
- The sugar detox plan is higher in healthy fats, organic when possible, colorful vegetables, and good source proteins. Natural fats make you feel full and satisfied, thus helping to reduce carb cravings.
- Eliminate all processed foods, refined sugars, and common food allergens such as commercial dairy, wheat/grains, soy, peanuts, and corn, as well as alcohol and caffeine.
- Add more colorful, local organic plant-based non-starchy carbs... VEGETABLES.
- Add more healthy fats to each meal like coconut oil, grass-fed butter, avocados, egg yolks, extra-virgin olive oil, MCT oil, raw nuts, and seeds

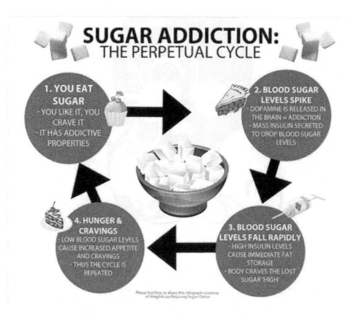

- Eat organic, grass fed, free roaming pasture protein
- Select raw nut butter except for peanuts. Unsalted and unroasted nuts.
- Avoid foods that cause inflammation to the body. Peanuts are high in omega 6 fatty acids which contribute to inflammation and inhibit recovery since we tend to be out of balance of omega three to six fatty acid ratio.
- No processed foods or refined sugars.
- No fruit allowed during this challenge as we eliminate sugars.
- Limit nuts - measure serving size ½ cup and put in a small bag. Eat only raw soaked nuts.
- No calorie counting required. Eat when you're hungry.
- No snacks are needed if you're eating balanced meals but eat a snack from the list if hungry; don't ever get to "hangry" (hungry + angry) or starving.
- High-fat diets will fill you up, and you will eat less plus feel satisfied and lose sugar cravings if not cheating yourself
- Replace one meal or snack per day (depending on activity level) with a good source grass-fed organic whey protein. Mix with water, ice, and healthy fats such as MCT oil or coconut milk.
- Follow the clean eating plan exactly as outlined for amazing results. If it is not on plan, don't eat or drink it – remember beverages and condiments add calories, sugar, sodium, etc.
- Remember, this is not a diet, but a JUMPSTART on a new eating lifestyle

Focus on eating these REAL Whole foods:

- Lots of organic, colorful, non-starchy vegetables
- Healthy fats such as avocado, coconut oil, ghee, fish oils, and grass-fed butter
- Wild caught fish such as salmon, trout, tuna, and mackerel
- Free range organic eggs including the egg yolk (fat soluble vitamins)
- Organic grass-fed meat free range and wild source
- Raw or low temperature processed sheep and goat dairy
- Raw nuts and seeds - unroasted
- Filtered or spring water with lemon, lime, or cucumber slices
- Probiotic foods as sauerkraut, kefir, and fermented foods

Before eating something, ask yourself...
- Are there less than five ingredients you can pronounce?
- Do you know what the ingredients are on the list?
- Does the food have an expiration date?
- Was the food around 10,000 years ago?

Avoid:
- Soy, Corn, Peanuts, Commercial Dairy (cow), Processed grains and gluten
- Alcohol
- Sugar and sugar substitutes
- Low-fat and non-fat processed foods
- Or limit caffeinated beverages (limit coffee to two cups per day; by noon)
- Processed, factory made, manufactured foods
- Excess calories from liquids and sugary drinks
- Factory-raised animal products
- Pesticide coated fruits and vegetables
- Vegetable oils including canola oil (excess omega 6s and inflammatory oils)
- Bottom-feeder fish (halibut, flounder, cod, shellfish, etc.)
- Pork
- Low-fat, non-fat, or diet products as they are very processed and usually high in carbohydrates
- Be aware of condiments and sauces as they usually contain sugar and unhealthy bad fats
- Limit your intake of processed vegetable and canola oils and mayonnaise.

- Limit alcohol because of the sugar or carbohydrates, as well as the connection to over-eating decisions, judgment, and poor sleep habits
- Sugar substitutes and sugar-free diet foods as they are not real food and usually highly processed
- High sugar foods: fruit juice, smoothies, cake, candy, etc.
- Fruit: if you need major reset eliminate for twenty-one days or try adding some local organic berries if in season and combine with fat/protein mix.
- Gluten and grains: wheat, rice, pasta, cereal, etc.
- Beans and legumes: kidney beans, lentils, peas, chickpeas
- Root vegetables: Potatoes, sweet potatoes, carrots, parsnips, etc. Unless you are participating in excess workouts.

Bottom Line: Avoid carb-based, processed foods including gluten, grains, sugars, legumes, candy, juice, and even most fruits. What are five foods and drinks you can eliminate today?

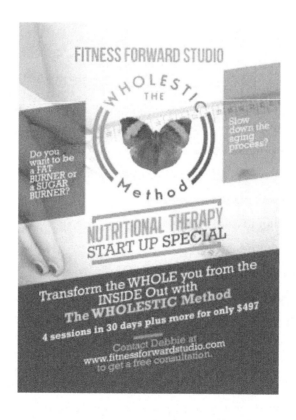

5-DAY JUMPSTART CHALLENGE MEAL PLAN AND RECIPES:

Daily Nutritional Shake: Add one packet of nutritional shake mix (I suggest WHOLE FOODS nutritional shake brand for my local clients) to one cup of clean source water. Shake in a shaker bottle or use a blender.

      a. Optional: if using a blender, add ice

      b. Optional: add one tablespoon chia seeds for fiber and omega 3 fatty acids

      c. If you need a more filling shake: add half a cup coconut milk

      d. Add new flavor: add cinnamon or one tablespoon raw organic nut butter

Clean Green Smoothie

2-4 celery stalks

1 cucumber

2-3 cups kale or chard

1-inch chunk of fresh ginger

1 lemon, juiced

1 tablespoon flaxseed oil or chia seeds

Water (or unsweetened almond, hemp, or coconut milk)

Green Goddess Smoothie

2-3 handfuls spinach

½ cucumber

½ avocado

1-2 stalks celery

1 tablespoon chia seeds

Water (or unsweetened almond, hemp, or coconut milk)

Green Monster:

3 large kale leaves

3-4 celery stalks

1/3 cucumber, peeled

1 lemon, peeled

1 handful of parsley

Fight & Repair Smoothie
Sliced ginger

1 lemon, sliced or juiced

1 teaspoon sliced turmeric

4 cups packed spinach and kale leaves

1 tablespoon Maca powder

1 tablespoon flaxseed oil-water

GI Healing Juice Recipe
½ head of cabbage

2 aloe leaves or 1 cup aloe juice

1 cucumber

1 tsp. fresh ginger

½ cup of peppermint leaves or pure extract

The WHOLE Athlete:
Cucumber, celery, kale, spinach, parsley, lemon,

Ginger, turmeric, and cayenne pepper and add collagen (find on my web page store).

Other good vegetables to blend or juice:
Base: celery, cucumber

Fiber: spinach, kale, parsley

Power Food add-ins: lemon, ginger, ginger, turmeric

Eliminate for now: apple, carrot, beet, orange

Add any of these foods to your green drink or super salad to detox the body plus many more options:

- Flaxseed oil
- Turmeric
- Olive oil
- Avocado oil
- Coconut oil
- Hemp oil
- Kale
- Spirulina
- Arugula
- Garlic

- Wheatgrass
- Spinach
- Lemons
- Limes
- Broccoli sprouts
- Onions

- Cabbage
- Brussels sprouts
- Blue-green algae
- Kelp
- Chard or Alfalfa sprouts

"Alternative Fuel:"

- Broccoli
- Cabbage
- Celery
- Cucumber
- Curly Parsley
- Lime
- Romaine Lettuce
- Wheat Grass
- Lemon
- Turmeric
- Kraut Juice
- Ginger
- Kale
- Spinach
- Parsley

The leaky gut syndrome is a rapidly growing condition that more and more people are struggling with every day. This condition may be the cause of your allergies, low energy, joint pain, autoimmune conditions, and weight gain. The GI Healing Juice recipe (listed above) will help repair your gut lining and decrease inflammation.

http://draxe.com/recipe/gi-healing-juice/
http://draxe.com/recipe/immune-boosting-juice/

> **For more green drink recipes and meal ideas sign up for my WHOLESTIC Method 5-Day Sugar Detox & Reset Jumpstart Challenge" board on Pinterest**
> **https://www.pinterest.com/WholesticMethod/**

Don't be afraid of consuming good essential fats that make you feel satisfied and full for hours, plus it helps you eat less.

5-DAY JUMPSTART CHALLENGE REAL FOOD MEAL IDEAS

Breakfast Anytime:
- 2-3 scrambled whole eggs
- Top with sliced avocado, salsa, or tomatoes and sautéed spinach (throw spinach over eggs when finished cooking).
- Cook eggs with coconut oil, Ghee, good source "Paleo" lard or quality bacon fat at medium heat.

Super Farm House Salad:
- Leafy green mix: kale, spinach, arugula (vegetables/carbs)
- Cut up cucumbers, celery, and yellow peppers (vegetables/carbs)
- Add 4-6 ounces grilled chicken, turkey, hardboiled eggs, or salmon (protein)
- Top with sliced avocado (¼ or ½ avocado) enough to keep full
- Top with EVOO and sea salt

Or... a large salad of mixed organic local leafy greens with chilled grilled organic vegetables such as yellow bell peppers, cucumber, tomatoes, and zucchini slices with a dash of sea salt and pepper and then top with avocado. Lightly sprinkle with raw macadamia nuts and olive oil.

Under the Sea:
- Grill or bake 4-6 ounces baked salmon or sea bass (wild) cooked with coconut oil
- Sauté or grill organic vegetables roasted in coconut oil – eat what is in season
- Topped with one tablespoon crushed, raw, unsalted, chopped nuts as pepitas (pumpkin seeds), almonds, or walnuts
- Option: add homemade pesto sauce by blending olive oil and basil in blender. Pesto includes blending pine nuts or cashews, salt, pepper, garlic. See ideas on my Pinterest boards.

Super bowl:
- 2-4 ounces organic chicken sausages (Whole Foods or local shop), grilled shrimp, or grilled scallops
- Shredded broccoli, cauliflower, and zucchini cooked in large pan with coconut oil or bacon fat
- Sauté raw, crushed walnuts in pan after vegetables out then use as topping
- Mix in bowl then top with sea salt and a drizzle of olive oil

Over the Rainbow Bowl of Goodness:
- Grill, broil, or sauté 2-4 ounces cod or halibut or other wild fish in season with coconut oil. Cook in pan then finish off in the oven for 5-7 minutes.
- In a big wok, cook 2-4 pieces of bacon, then remove bacon from pan
- Sauté 1-2 plus cups of chopped or sliced Brussels sprouts in the bacon fat. Remove to side (try food processor for slicing Brussels sprouts)
- Cook crushed walnuts or macadamia nuts in pan
- Mix the Brussels sprouts and bacon together
- Serve fish over bed of Brussels sprouts mix then top with roasted nuts
- Add tablespoon of grass-fed butter on top for more taste or if dry (Kerry Gold)

Morning Choices:

IF DOING COFFEE: Exdrogenous Ketones Fat Coffee or a type of "Bullet Proof" coffee: this is coffee blended with one tablespoon coconut oil or MCT oil and one tablespoon of grass-fed butter - Kerry Gold Butter. Optional: add cinnamon. Use a blender for best mixing for buttery fat filling coffee. Use French press at home. Great for a busy morning or before a long training ride, hike, or run, if metabolically efficient. Or use Exdrogenous Ketone supplement with your favorite herbal tea. Pruvit or Perfect Keto are good options for supplement ketones.

Morning Power Smoothie: use shake mix provided with one cup of water. Optional added healthy fats to make more filling: add one tablespoon MCT oil or half a cup real, unsweetened, full-fat coconut milk (see Amazon.com links). You can add one tablespoon of chia seeds, one cup of organic spinach, kale, or greens mix if you need more vegetables and nutrients.

Emergency Backup Snacks: Remember: if eating a higher fat, low carb food plan, you should be satisfied ("full") for three plus hours. Keep track of emotions, where you are eating, why you are eating, and level of hunger in your food logs. No snacking or emotional eating, but you should not feel starving or "hangry."

- Vegetable crudités as celery, cucumber, yellow pepper, and jicama.
- Raw, unsalted almonds, macadamia nuts, or cashews, but measure half a cup into bag
- Hardboiled eggs from good source
- Green vegetable juice: kale, spinach, celery, cucumber, lemon, or other varieties.
- Rollups: 2-4 ounces sliced grass fed organic turkey with raw goat or sheep cheese slices if doing dairy for 5-Day challenge
- Celery sticks with almond butter or cashew butter
- Cucumber, celery, red pepper with freshly made guacamole (avocado w/Pico)
- Olives and pickles from the olive bar

Healthy fats:
- saturated fats as lard, tallow, chicken fat, duck fat, goose fat, clarified butter/ghee, butter, coconut oil, MCT oil
- monounsaturated fats like avocado, macadamia and olive oil
- polyunsaturated omega 3s, especially from animal sources (fatty fish, seafood)
- coconut and olives

Grass-fed and wild animal sources:
- grass-fed meat (beef, lamb, goat, venison)

- wild-caught fish and seafood (avoid farmed fish)
- pastured pork and poultry (free range)
- pastured eggs, gelatin, ghee, butter
- offal, grass-fed (liver, heart, kidneys, and other organ meats)

Non-starchy vegetables:

- Organic leafy greens: spinach, kale, arugula, butter lettuce, Swiss chard, bok choy, spinach, lettuce, chard, chives, endive, radicchio, etc.
- Organic cruciferous vegetables as kohlrabi, radishes
- Celery stalk, asparagus, cucumber, summer squash, zucchini, spaghetti squash, yellow and orange peppers
- Occasionally add some cruciferous vegetables (white and green cabbage, red cabbage, cauliflower, broccoli, Brussels sprouts, fennel, turnips, rutabaga/swede)

Fruits:

- avocados
- tomatoes

Condiments:

- Real mustard- no sugar on label
- Homemade pesto
- Bone broth
- Pickles – no sugar added
- Fermented foods: kimchi, kombucha, and sauerkraut (read labels - no sugar)
- All spices and herbs, lemon or lime juice, and zest
- Grass-fed natural plain whey protein
- Collagen: (grass-fed, hormone free)

Vegetables, Mushrooms, and Fruits: *eat occasionally after 5-Day Jumpstart Challenge:*

- nightshades (eggplant, tomatoes, peppers)
- some root vegetables (parsley root), spring onion, leek, onion, garlic, mushrooms, winter squash (pumpkin)
- okra, bean sprouts, sugar snap peas, wax beans, globe or French artichokes, water chestnuts
- berries after the 5-Day Jumpstart Challenge are allowed as (blackberries, blueberries, strawberries, raspberries, cranberries, mulberries, etc.

Grain-fed animal sources and full-fat raw dairy:

- beef, poultry, eggs, and ghee (avoid farmed pork - toxic and high in omega 6)
- local raw goat or sheep cheese
- After twenty-one days, if okay with dairy, add plain full-fat yogurt, cottage cheese, cream, sour cream, cheese (avoid products labeled low-fat or non-fat)
- Bacon – only from good source nitrate free, no added preservatives, or sugar

Nuts and seeds:

- macadamia nuts (very low in carbs, high in omega 3s)
- raw seeds to soak - chia seeds, hemp seeds, flax seeds
- raw, unroasted nuts - almonds, cashews, pecans, walnuts, hazelnuts, Brazil, etc.
- Seeds as pumpkin seeds, sesame seeds, or sunflower seeds

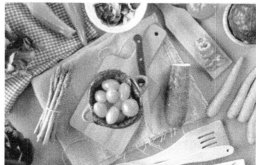

Fermented Foods:

- Fermented soy as Tempeh, Natto, soy sauce or coconut aminos
- Sauerkraut
  Pickles (no sugar) and sea vegetables as nori and kombu

Dessert:

If you need a sweet treat, try my Chia seed pudding by mixing ½ cup of chia seeds with one cup of water. Let it sit and then mix together. Once you have a pudding consistency add your toppings. Blend one tablespoon coconut flakes (unsweetened), raw unsalted almond butter, and cinnamon or just mix a spoonful of raw almond butter and coconut oil in ramekin size dish.

If you haven't already set up our The WHOLESTIC Method text messaging service - get started by texting the word THEWHOLEATHLETE to the number 31996 today.

THE WHOLESTIC METHOD
5-DAY JUMPSTART DETOX & RESET CHALLENGE
DAILY ACCOUNTABILITY REPORT

Date: _____

Rate on your day today: 1-5 (5 being best)

1   2   3   4   5

Please answer these questions daily: be honest:

1. Did you replace a meal a day with our Nutritional Shake and add healthy fat as coconut milk, flax oil or MCT C8 brain oil?

   ❑ Yes   ❑ No

2. How was your energy level today? _____

   _____
   _____

3. How were your cravings for sugar, alcohol, or other vices?

   _____
   _____
   _____

4. Did you eat when you were hungry?

   ❑ Yes   ❑ No

5. How long were you full and satisfied for after you shake or meal?

   _____

6. Did you need a snack today because you were hungry? ❑ Yes   ❑ No

7. Did you sleep 7-9 hours last night? Bed by 10:00 p.m.?

   ❑ Yes   ❑ No

8. Did you work out today and what did you do? (3 x strength workouts/week) ❑ Yes   ❑ No

9. Goals achieved today?

   a. _____

      b. _____

      c. _____

10. Any struggles, challenges, or areas of opportunity that you can approach differently to improve tomorrow?

      a. _____

      b. _____

List your goals for tomorrow including elements included in The WHOLESTIC Method: food, exercise, sleep, stress, movement, digestion health, hydration, and happiness?

1. _____

2. _____

3. _____

THE WHOLESTIC METHOD ACCOUNTABILITY REPORT: DAY ONE

1. How are you feeling? How are your moods, energy level, and cravings?

2. How is your sleep?

3. Are you hydrating throughout the day and retaining water (not coming out the other end)?

4. How is your ACV detox drink each day?

5. Gut health? Bloated belly, inflammation, gas, indigestion, reflux?

   - Most of the bloating will go away because you are giving up sugar. That's a big step and a big win.

   - We know sugar feeds all kinds of possible yeasts and pathogens that may have in the small intestine.

- Removing sugar from a food for these parasites can greatly diminish symptoms of dysbiosis such as bloating.

6. *Nutritional Therapy Functional Evaluation*: I can test the tenderness (score) of the Chapman Stomach Duodenum reflex with ACV as the digestive and see if the score dropped. We would also be very interested in the Bennett's Reflex points for the small intestine and find if much inflammation in the gut.

7. The FE will tell us the true story of how well ACV detox drink or any digestive aid put in place is working or not working well enough to support HCL sufficiency as an important phase of digestion from North to South.

Detox drink tip:

- Adding ACV to a small amount of water before a meal will temporarily increase the acidity of the stomach, but it does not increase HCL production. The drawback to this method is that too often people take too much water to get the ACV down the hatch and end up diluting the already insufficient HCL they have and make matters worse.

- I can test your stomach acid and stomach-duodenum reflex points to see if you are deficient in HCL acid (stomach acid), which is essential for proper digestion and absorbing nutrients. If you are opposed to trying Betaine or another HCL supplement, you can try three teaspoons of ACV with no more than three teaspoons of water. You could also add digestive bitters to the ACV concoction for better results. Digestive Bitters tap into the body's neuro-lingual response that occurs when you taste something bitter. The bitter taste stimulates increased stomach acid production, as well as other digestive juices.

LET ME KNOW YOUR UPDATE, PROGRESS, AND AH-HA'S SO FAR THIS WEEK- SHARE THEM ON OUR FACEBOOK PAGE- THE WHOLESTIC METHOD 5-DAY JUMPSTART CHALLENGE.

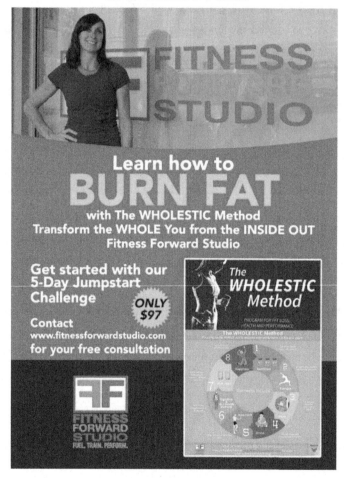

THE 5-DAY JUMPSTART CHALLENGE: DAY TWO DAILY ACCOUNTABILITY HOMEWORK REPORT:

1. How did you feel this morning?
2. *Weight from Monday morning?* Don't weigh in again until next Friday or the weekend.
3. *Daily Goals:* What are your goals today based on yesterday?
4. Poop check... how many times per day do you poop? Sign of digestive health.
5. Homework today: listen to this podcast we did on digestion health and your poop. Let me know what you learned from the episode. Download from this link on my web page or find on iTunes - "The WHOLE Athlete" podcast by Debbie Potts.
6. http://tinyurl.com/PoopyPolice

Daily Accountability Report: due at the end of the day by 8:00 p.m.
1. Nutrition: What did you eat today? As per the plan.

   _____
   _____
   _____
   _____

2. Exercise: what was your workout today?

   _____
   _____
   _____
   _____
   _____

3. Sleep: hours slept? Time to bed?

   _____ _____

4. Stress level: Scale 1-10 (10 max stress Gut symptoms?

   _____

_____

5. Hydration: Did you drink half of your body weight in ounces of water today?
    ☐ Yes   ☐ No

6. Happiness: Did you write three things you were grateful for today before bed?

    _____

    _____

    _____

    _____

Get your mind right. It is game time. If you did not already turn in the forms, please find them all on my website - links for new client forms on the top banner:

http://debbiepotts.net/phase-one-5-day-jumpstart

Please answer the following questions that will aid with your individual weekly goals:
1. What is your motivation for doing the program?
2. What would you like to learn or accomplish in this next week?

Your daily accountability homework report overview for the next 5-plus days: How did you do and feel today? Reflect on how you really feel from the inside out.

Review what you learned about The WHOLESTIC Method eight elements:
1. Nutrition: What did you eat today? _____

    _____

    _____

2. Exercise: What was your workout today? _____

    _____

    _____

3. Sleep: How many hours did you sleep? _____ What time did you go to bed? _____

4. Stress level: Scale 1-10 (10 max stress) _____

5. Movement: How many steps do you take per day? _____ How many every hour? _____

6. Digestion: Did you take a probiotic? _____ What are your gut symptoms? _____

    _____

7. Hydration: Did you drink half your body weight in ounces of water? Yes _____ No _____

8. Happiness: Did you write/journal three things you were grateful for today before bed? Yes _____ No _____

THE WHOLESTIC METHOD DETOX & RESET ACCOUNTABILITY REPORT

(Used for 5-Day Jumpstart Challenge)

Rate yourself 1-5 (5 being best)

1   2   3   4   5

Name: _____

Date: _____

Starting Weight: _____

Body Fat Percentage: _____

Ending Weight: _____

Date: _____

Ending Body Fat Percentage: _____

Did you replace a meal a day with our nutritional shake?

❑ Yes   ❑ No

Did you make one green drink or buy one at Juju Beet?

❑ Yes   ❑ No

Did you sleep seven to nine hours a night for all five days?

❑ Yes   ❑ No

Did you work out five times per week for the five days hard/easy days?

❑ Yes   ❑ No

Did you earn over 100 MEPs per workout with your MYZONE belt?

❑ Yes   ❑ No

Did you drink half your body weight in ounces of water throughout the day?

❑ Yes   ❑ No

Did you move 10,000 steps per day?

❑ Yes   ❑ No

Did you write in your gratitude journal each night?

❑ Yes   ❑ No

Goal Achieved?

❑ Yes   ❑ No

Next Step/Suggestions: _____

_____

_____

_____

Sit with your assigned fitness coach to review your scorecard results and start your phase two program:

http://thewholesticmethod.com

THE WHOLESTIC METHOD
5-DAY JUMPSTART CHALLENGE DAILY JOURNAL
REPORT #1: DAY ONE

Congratulations. Your first day of the 5-Day Jumpstart Challenge is complete...almost. Now it is time to start completing your daily journal to stay accountable and committed to the process.

Reminders:

- No eating after 8:00 p.m. so make sure you finish your meal or shake at least two hours before bed. The kitchen is CLOSED after your last meal.
- Goal to not eat again for 12-15 hours for a natural type of fast.
- Send your accountability report to your team or your coach
- Also, I am working on doing more cooking and exercise videos on my YouTube Channel if you need ideas and workouts... subscribe then you get the updates: https://www.youtube.com/c/fitforwardbellevue/videos

Date: _____

Pick three goals for the next day:

1._____

2._____

3._____

Daily Tracking:

EXERCISE: What was your workout today? _____

_____

_____

MOVEMENT:

How many hours were you idle today? _____

(Get up every hour)

Total Steps today? _____

Supplements: _____

Food goals today? _____

SLEEP:

What time did you go to bed last night? _____

Wake up this morning? _____

How was your sleep quality? ____Sound ____Restless

Did you awake during the night? ____Yes ____No

How many times? _____

Reasons why? _____

Did you have night sweats? ____ Yes ____No

Did you wake up refreshed today or tired?

____ Refreshed ____ Tired

Did you start slow this morning? ____ Yes ____No

If yes, how long did it take you to feel alert? _____

_____

DIGESTION: Bowel movements?

Number: _____Color: _____

Size & Shape: _____

STRESS: Heart Rate Variability Score: _____

What are three things you are grateful for today?

1. _____

2. _____

3. _____

Example of my personal daily accountability report:

I ate a big meal at 3:30 p.m. and just finished work. I won't eat when I get home and going to bed but 8:00 p.m. I am lifting weights tomorrow morning and running thirty minutes at 11:30 a.m.

I want you to not only evaluate your day, but also determine what your goals are for the next day. Based on what your areas of opportunities are from your experience. Make sure you schedule in your workouts for the week. If you have a busy work day, you need to get up and get outside for a thirty-minute walk before your day begins.

Drink your one to two glasses of clean water with Himalayan sea salt first thing in the morning. Throughout the day, you should be drinking the "secret detox drink" that is in the manual. Apple cider vinegar or lemon juice and cayenne pepper in your water bottle.

THE WHOLESTIC METHOD 5-DAY JUMPSTART CHALLENGE DAILY JOURNAL
REPORT #2: DAY TWO

Here is your reading homework today...

1. As we eliminate gluten. Where is gluten hiding?
   Read this blog: http://draxe.com/recipe/secret-detox-drink
2. Complete daily accountability report each day to keep on track
3. Add more fat to your nutrition shake (coconut milk, MCT oil, half an avocado or one tablespoon raw almond butter)
4. Complete your metabolic type questionnaire and health appraisal form.
5. Did you get your starting weight yesterday?

Daily Accountability Report: due at the end of the day by 8:00 p.m.

Questions for you today:

1. How did you feel this morning?
2. *Weight from Monday morning?*
3. *Daily Goals:* What are your goals today based on yesterday?
4. Poop check... how many times per day do you poop? Sign of digestive health.
5. Homework: Download from this link on my web page or find on iTunes The WHOLE Athlete podcast by Debbie Potts. Search for statin drug and cholesterol episodes
6. Nutrition: What did you eat today? _____
   _____
   _____
7. Exercise: What was your workout today? _____
   _____
   _____
8. Sleep: How many hours did you sleep? _____ What time did you go to bed? _____

9. Stress level: Scale 1-10 (10 max stress) _____

10. Movement: How many steps do you take per day? _____ How many every hour? _____

11. Digestion: Did you take a probiotic? _____ What are your gut symptoms? _____

_____

12. Hydration: Did you drink half your body weight in ounces of water? Yes _____ No _____

13. Happiness: Did you write/journal three things you were grateful for today before bed? Yes _____ No _____

THE WHOLESTIC METHOD
5-DAY JUMPSTART DAILY JOURNAL
REPORT #3: DAY THREE

Daily Accountability Report: due at the end of the day by 8:00 p.m.

Questions for you today:

1. How did you feel this morning?
2. *Weight from Monday morning?*
3. *Daily Goals:* What are your goals today based on yesterday?
4. Poop check… how many times per day do you poop? Sign of digestive health.
5. Homework: Download from this link on my web page or find on iTunes The WHOLE Athlete podcast by Debbie Potts. Search for statin drug and cholesterol episodes
6. Nutrition: What did you eat today? _____

   _____

   _____
7. Exercise: What was your workout today? _____

   _____

   _____
8. Sleep: How many hours did you sleep? _____ What time did you go to bed? _____
9. Stress level: Scale 1-10 (10 max stress) _____
10. Movement: How many steps do you take per day? _____ How many every hour? _____
11. Digestion: Did you take a probiotic? _____ What are your gut symptoms? _____

    _____
12. Hydration: Did you drink half your body weight in ounces of water? Yes _____ No _____
13. Happiness: Did you write/journal three things you were grateful for today before bed? Yes _____ No _____

THE WHOLESTIC METHOD
5-DAY JUMPSTART CHALLENGE DAILY JOURNAL
REPORT #4: DAY FOUR

Day Four is here... one day left, and then you progress to the 21-day challenge which is continuing to eat no sugar or grains. Please complete and send back your Daily Accountability Report.

Here is your homework today:

1. How was your heart rate test yesterday? Try it after eating a food you feel like you may have a sensitivity to base on post-meal symptoms.

   Let's talk about glycemic index and which vegetables and carbs are best to eat. When you gradually add carbohydrates into your food plan (80/20 program), then you can learn which is the best type as well as always combining an organic non-GMO carbohydrate with a healthy fat and grass-fed protein. Of course, ignore eating the processed foods and sugary foods on this list... just learn more about the vegetables you eat (carrots versus cucumber) and when you re-introduce fruit to your diet.

   See more on: http://www.glycemicedge.com/glycemic-index-chart

   Glycemic Food List
   "With the Glycemic Index (GI), it's all about the quality of carbohydrates, not the quantity (though, if you want to include both GI and quantity, you should stick with GL foods of < 20). If you're just getting started on the GI diet, you may want to print or link (below) to this reference. Understanding how your body breaks down carbs and the impact of blood sugar and subsequent counter-acting release of insulin is the very core of the glycemic index process. For a quick recap of how blood sugar interactions work, be sure to read our tutorial and learn how and why these are important."
   - **High GI Foods** = GI of 70+ (Try to avoid.)
   - **Medium GI** = 55 – 69 (use caution.)
   - **Low GI** = 0 – 54 (This is your target zone, look for foods with a low GI

260

score)

"Many nutritionists prefer to look at the Glycemic Load (GL) rather than just the Glycemic Index (GI) for individual foods. That's because the load of a food also incorporates the quantity of carbs per serving. They're both simple scores you can look for, so it's easy to get started."

2. Read: http://tinyurl.com/11DaysGlutFree

3. Find the episodes on ketogenic, low carb, saturated fats, and cholesterol. Search for various episodes by searching on the "feed" section on iTunes or on podcast tab on my website - see podcast archives.

4. How are you feeling? Any detox symptoms or sugar withdrawals? Are you eating low carb of 100 grams or less per day?
   - Drink more water through the day. Pack a bottle for your car and work.
   - Also, add more fat with your meals especially if you need a snack.
   - If busy and low energy... have another shake. You can buy more at Whole Foods.

Daily Accountability Report: due at the end of the day by 8:00 p.m.

Questions for you today:
1. How did you feel this morning?
2. *Weight from Monday morning?*
3. *Daily Goals:* What are your goals today based on yesterday?
4. Poop check... how many times per day do you poop? Sign of digestive health.
5. Homework: Download from this link on my web page or find on iTunes The WHOLE Athlete podcast by Debbie Potts. Search for statin drug and cholesterol episodes
6. Nutrition: What did you eat today? _____
   _____
   _____
7. Exercise: What was your workout today? _____
   _____
   _____
8. Sleep: How many hours did you sleep? _____ What time did you go to bed? _____

9. Stress level: Scale 1-10 (10 max stress) _____

10. Movement: How many steps do you take per day? _____ How many every hour? _____

11. Digestion: Did you take a probiotic? _____ What are your gut symptoms? _____

_____

12. Hydration: Did you drink half your body weight in ounces of water? Yes _____ No _____

13. Happiness: Did you write/journal three things you were grateful for today before bed? Yes _____ No _____

THE WHOLESTIC METHOD PHASE ONE 5-DAY JUMPSTART CHALLENGE DAILY JOURNAL
REPORT #5: DAY FIVE

Here is your homework today:

1. Homework: The Four Food Devils by Paul Chek. Read blog at http://tinyurl.com/5StepNoDetox

2. Remember to eat right for your metabolic type or even try eating per blood type. If you eat the right ratio of fat/protein/carbs, you should be feeling energetic twenty minutes after eating - not sluggish or tired. Evaluate how you feel after you eat today...

3. <u>The Four Food Devils</u>: We have eliminated this four "devils" during our jumpstart, and we will continue to eliminate them from our daily food plan. Certain "non-foods" as these "devils" will cause you to feel tired, lethargic and depressed per Paul Chek - they take more energy out of the body to break down or process than the nutrition they provide the body with nourishment. Most of these four devils, as we discussed in the manual, create inflammation in the body including digestion, joint, muscular, energy and mood issues.

   They are:
   - Processed pasteurized dairy
   - Table salt- sodium chloride
   - White sugar
   - White flour

<u>Daily Accountability Report: due at the end of the day by 8:00 p.m.</u>

Questions for you today:

1. Nutrition: What did you eat today? As per the plan.

   _____

   _____

   _____

   _____

2. Exercise: what was your workout today?

_____

_____

_____

_____

3. Sleep: hours slept? Time to bed?

    _____   _____

4. Stress level: Scale 1-10 (10 max stress Gut symptoms?

    _____

    _____

    _____

    _____

5. Hydration: Did you drink half of your body weight in ounces of water today?
    ❑ Yes   ❑ No

6. Happiness: Did you write three things you were grateful for today before bed?

    _____

    _____

    _____

    _____

    _____

THE WHOLESTIC METHOD 5-DAY JUMPSTART DETOX & RESET CHALLENGE SUMMARY:

1. Complete the metabolic type form and health appraisal form for your information. Then, highlight the areas you scored on (health form) to focus on improving or figuring out your "Why."

2. The links to the forms are on www.debbiepotts.net

3. The Daily Accountability email examples are in the upcoming section. These are sent out to clients each day during the program with reminders, tips, tricks, and homework.

4. Keep it simple...NO SUGAR and NO GRAINS.

5. Drink fresh, organic, vegetable-green juice drinks, plus your detox drink, herbal detox tea, and water with sea salt.

6. Eat one big meal per day late afternoon or early evening = higher healthy fats, moderate protein, and low carbohydrate (vegetables).

7. Follow your metabolic type (see forms on the website) to determine the best ratio of macronutrients. Most people do best on a lower carb, higher fat real food plan, but your body will tell you if you are eating right for your type. You should feel energized within twenty minutes after your meal and satisfied for three or more hours (or longer if a fat burner).

8. Snack if you're hungry. See food list for ideas (low carb ideas that will fill you up and keep you full longer). Gradually, you will not need to snack as you become a fat burner and get off the blood sugar roller coaster.

9. Drink one shake (or two if more active) with water and add a healthy fat—such as coconut milk or nut butter—to keep yourself more satiated.

10. See rest of guidelines in the manual for exercise, sleep, stress, digestion, movement, and happiness

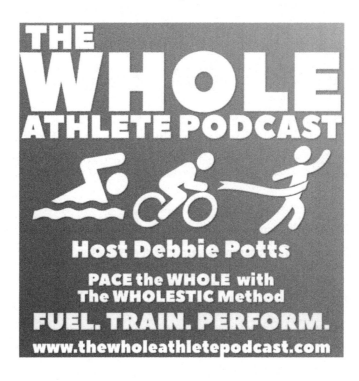

Great job in completing your first 5-Day Jumpstart Challenge!

Congratulations for following Phase One of The WHOLESTIC Method program, as well as sticking to the stricter guidelines for your 5-Day Jumpstart Challenge.

Day Five is here... here is some homework for you...

1. Let's learn more about our gut *health, digestion, and the brain...* the vagal nerve connects the gut and brain. Remember when you get nervous (the brain) and then you often get butterflies in your tummy (gut)? Listen to my weekly podcast to learn more!
    a. Digestion impacts the entire body, as well as the other foundation pillars in nutritional therapy: digestion, blood sugar handling, essential fatty acids, minerals, and hydration.
    b. http://articles.mercola.com/sites/articles/archive/2016/01/07/how-gut-microbiome-influences-health.aspx

2. *The benefits of apple cider vinegar*
    a. https://authoritynutrition.com/6-proven-health-benefits-of-apple-cider-vinegar/

3. **What is next after the 5-Day Jumpstart Challenge?**
   a. Keep at it, but add more real food. Continue adding healthier natural fats, proteins, and vegetables while avoiding sugar and grains.
   b. Tomorrow – keep on the "NSNG" "JERF" food plan which means eating whole foods without a label of manufactured ingredients and fillers. Eat low carb, moderate protein, and higher healthy fats.
   c. I know some of you want to drink alcohol tomorrow, but try your best to stay on the detox program – for sure on the weekdays and don't blow it on the weekends by overindulging. Keep hydrating and using the detox drink each day.

4. Send me your week ***review and testimonial*** to add to our website for The WHOLESTIC Method 5-day Jumpstart Sugar Detox & Reset Challenge. Send via www.debbiepotts.net. I know you probably have a few questions as we work to move forward with keeping up these new "The WHOLESTIC Method" habits after your experience last week. Please turn in your accountability reports from last week as well as your final review, weight loss, evaluation of your transformation experience and a testimonial you would love to share the website.

Below are common questions:

1. **Is it okay to add coffee back in tomorrow?**
   a. Listen to your body, your heart rate, and response to drinking coffee
   b. If it's okay, then make sure you drink an organic source
   c. Limit coffee to two cups in the day - ideally before noon.
   d. Drink herbal tea instead

2. **What about legumes?**
   a. Legumes have a lot of carbohydrates
   b. If eating legume, you must soak them for proper digestions and to release the phytic acid:
      - *"Like grains and pseudo grains, legumes contain phytic acid. Phytic acid binds to nutrients in the food, preventing you from absorbing them. It doesn't steal any nutrients that are already in your body, but it does make that bowl of lentils a lot less nutrient-dense than the Nutrition Facts panel would have you believe."*

- *http://www.westonaprice.org/beginner-videos/proper-preparation-of-grains-and-legumes-video-by-sarah-pope/*
- http://paleoleap.com/beans-and-legumes/

3. *How often should one continue with the detox drink? Daily?*
   a. I believe in having the APC drink almost daily, as well as the detox tea (Yogi brand is good)
   b. We live in a toxic world – every day and everywhere we are surrounded by toxins. We eat them, breathe them, and put them on our skin.
   c. Read more: http://fitnessforwardstudio.com/the-wholestic-method/links/

4. *Are root vegetables okay to add in?*
   a. Watch the carbohydrates and glycemic index. Hopefully, you did the metabolic typing questionnaire via the website links and learned if you can tolerate carbohydrates or not
   b. Make sure you eat carbohydrates with healthy fats and protein, but for sure with healthy fat to slow absorption, add flavor and satiety.

5. *What about fruits?*
   a. Make sure you don't eat fruit without also eating a fat and protein or, at least, fats to slow absorption as the goal is to balance our blood sugar levels
   b. See glycemic index charts or books for lists of best organic sources

6. *Should you continue to stay off dairy?*
   Here are great examples of easy-to-read blogs to follow:
   - https://draxe.com/recipe/secret-detox-drink/
   - Chris Kressor
   - Dr. Mercola

And now, to the details of the next phase!

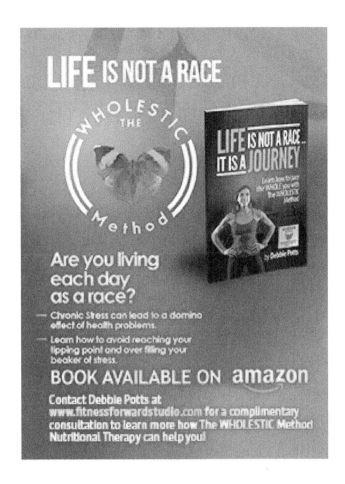

WHAT IS YOUR NEXT STEP TO BECOMING A WHOLESTIC ATHLETE?

Download and subscribe to my podcast on iTunes, The WHOLE Athlete, or find past episodes on www.thewholeathletepodcast.com.

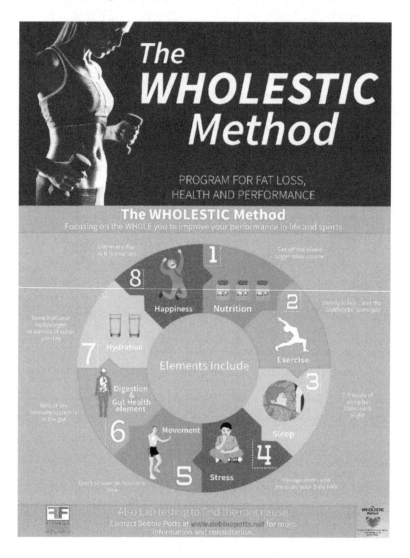

Now, what is the next step? Keep reading for your maintenance stage.

STEP #5
PHASE TWO:
THE 21-DAY DETOX & RESET CHALLENGE

Now that you have completed the 5-Day Jumpstart Challenge, don't go crazy. Move to Phase Two. The next 21-plus days will teach you the tools to become a fat burning machine with our WHOLE person approach.

Are you ready to look and feel amazing on the inside and out and get off the blood sugar roller coaster?

The WHOLESTIC Method 21-Day Challenge is more than just another weight loss or detox program designed to help you lose weight by changing the way you eat. You will start a new journey as you begin to teach your body how to use fat as the main fuel source and have less reliance on sugar as we focus on the other elements of transforming into a new improved you from the inside out with The WHOLESTIC Method.

My approach is unique because we are not only going to eliminate foods that create chaos in your body, but we will also work on exercise, sleep, stress, movement, digestions, hydration, and most importantly for fat loss and health... your happiness.

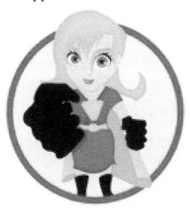

I would suggest not going overboard through the weekend and self-sabotaging the gains and progress you've made during your "detox & reset" challenge. Keep in mind, the benefits of eating healthy fats with your meals helps balance blood sugar. That includes drinking alcohol.

Speaking of alcohol, I know lots of you enjoy drinking in the evenings and weekends. I would **love** for you to review the last week of not drinking and determine your "WHY?" *Why* do you need a drink after work or in the evening with dinner? *Why* do you need to drink to relax instead of going for an evening walk? *Why* do you feel the urge to have alcohol at all? Enjoy the weekend while you continue to eat real food and add in more meals instead of a shake. Let me know how you are doing and feeling... plus did you weigh-in today after your 5-day detox and reset challenge? I suggest weighing in once a week as we are working on creating new habits and improve our mindset, so don't obsess about the scale weight.

Something you can do over the weekend is to write up a review, feedback, or testimonial so I can improve the program in the future. I would suggest finding a Nutritional Therapy Practitioner near you to really transform the WHOLE you from the inside out. I am committed to inspire others to live by 'The WHOLESTIC Method.'

So, let's get started on what you should focus on these next three weeks as you move forward with your fat loss and reset challenge. The Phase One program was a little more challenging, but it sets you up for success on Phase Two as we start the 21-day challenge to continue working on breaking the sugar addiction and resetting our habits from the eight elements of The WHOLESTIC Method. This program will help you burn fat, optimize your total health and improve your performance in daily life as you make the transition off the blood sugar roller coaster as well as supporting your adrenals, digestion and gut health!

Stay away from... or limit to 80% of the time:

- Soy, Corn, Peanuts, and Commercial Dairy (cow)
- Alcohol
- Sugar and sugar substitute
- Gluten and processed grains
- Low-fat and non-fat processed foods
- Caffeine
- Processed manufactured foods
- Excess calories from liquids

- Factory raised animal products
- Pesticide coated fruits and vegetables
- Vegetable oils including Canola oil
- Bottom feeder fish
- Pork

REMEMBER: Foods to Reduce or Avoid: Think no evil whites and low carb for the 21 days or more:

1. Avoid low-fat, non-fat, or diet products as they are very processed and high in carbohydrates.
2. Be aware of condiments and sauces as they contain sugar and unhealthy, bad fats.
3. Avoid or limit your intake of processed vegetable oils and mayonnaise, including canola oil.
4. Avoid or limit alcohol because of the sugar or carbohydrates as well as the connection to overeating decisions, judgment, and poor sleep habits.
5. Avoid sugar substitutes and sugar-free diet foods as they are not real food and highly-processed.
6. Avoid high sugar foods: fruit juice, smoothies, cake, candy, etc.
7. Limit or avoid fruit: if you need major reset eliminate for 21 days or try adding some local organic berries if in season and combine with fat/protein mix.
8. Avoid gluten and grains: wheat, rice, pasta, cereal and more
9. Avoid beans and legumes: kidney beans, lentils, peas, chickpeas
10. Avoid root vegetables: Potatoes, sweet potatoes, carrots, parsnips, etc. - unless you are participating in excess workouts.

Your plate will vary based on what works best for your metabolic type but here is one example of a low carb, moderate protein and higher healthy fat meal plan that is beneficial if metabolically damaged and other diseases as auto-immune issues.

Timing Guidelines

Suggestions for Becoming Fat Adapted:

- Eat last meal three to four hours prior to bedtime
- Wait upon waking to eat when you're hungry.
- As you become fat adapted, you will be less hungry as we are training our body to utilize fat as your main go-to fuel source and not rely on sugar (at rest and low-intensity exercise).
- You will reduce your hunger levels and sugar cravings by eating whole foods that leave you full and satisfied.
- Once a week, try a 5-17 hour fast (if not stressed) by stopping eating after dinner, and waiting to eat breakfast (Intermittent Fasting)
- Adding more essential fats to your diet will keep you full and satisfied for hours.

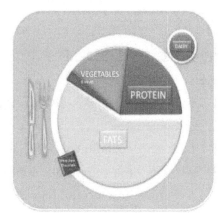

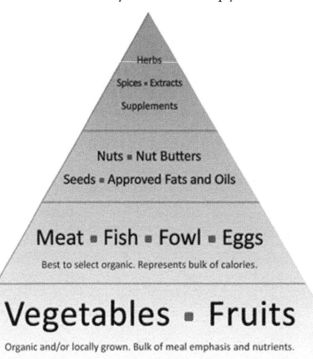

Now, you wonder what you should eat every day? It's simple once you get started and think outside the box of the eating the Standard American Diet (S.A.D.) I enjoy eating fresh vegetables (salads) every day, and I prepare meals that take less than ten minutes (or my husband cooks for me). You will find your favorite meal plans as you experiment with mixing real food ingredients as well as reading many of the great real food cookbooks available on Amazon or your local bookstore.

One of my favorite books is by Diane Sanfilippo, *Practical Paleo*, as well as her Sugar Detox cookbooks. Both are easy to follow and have great pictures. Also, see Mark Sisson's *Primal Blueprint* cookbook and Anna Vocino's *Eat Happy* no sugar or grains cookbook. Bonus: follow me on Pinterest and Instagram for more of my favorite's meal ideas on:

http://tinyurl.com/WHOLESTICMethodSugarDetox

For great ideas on becoming a WHOLE Athlete and fat burning machine with my WHOLESTIC Method program.

Remember, you don't need to have an S.A.D. breakfast as toast, oatmeal, cereal, and juice. This is exactly what you don't want. Why not try lunch foods for breakfast? Eat when hungry and stop when full. Reprogram your mindset that you need to eat the S.A.D. for each meal. Instead, eat a plant-based diet matched with healthy proteins and fats in the right amount for you.

Listen to your body and the signals after meals as your body will tell you what is too much or too little. You should be energized after you eat and satisfied for at least three or four hours or else you may have gut issues, food sensitivities, and/or an imbalance of nutrients for your metabolic type.

My eating schedule and habits:

My weekday schedule is different than most people, as most my work day is 5:00-11:30 a.m., then often another shift from 3:30–7:00 p.m. Based on my work and training schedule as well as my Metabolic Type (Protein), I tend to eat one larger meal in the afternoon with the correct blend of macronutrients that keeps me full for hours. I am only full and satisfied if I eat for my metabolic type (higher fat/protein mix with vegetables). I try to avoid eating a meal too close to bedtime (7:30-8:00 p.m.), or else I feel uncomfortable going to bed with a full belly. If I am feeling hungry in the evening, I will have a small snack of healthy fats, protein, and maybe some vegetables. The trick is to listen to your body when you are full and satisfied and eat right for your type to avoid overeating and binging.

Another tip: the kitchen is closed after 8:00 p.m.

275

I am fortunate to be married to someone who is an amazing chef as all I am good at preparing are salads, vegetable trays, and chia seed pudding. On weekends, my husband and I usually have dinner with friends one night, but I prefer his cooking over eating out; plus, we can control how the food is cooked prepared. We cook with good quality bacon fat we save from cooking or use organic coconut oil. I use olive oil for salads and cooked vegetables with a sprinkle of Himalayan sea salt.

Breakfast can be for dinner or eat dinner leftovers for lunch, as needed. If you eat too many carbs or sugar for your metabolic type, then you probably will feel more tired, fatigued, and craving more sweets.

Plan the night, especially if heading to work or going off to a busy full scheduled day or event. Personally, I don't have time for a sit-down breakfast meal most days of the week if my schedule is packed with client sessions. I need to go for the liquid fat calories (not ideal, but depends on your work schedule) of Bullet Proof coffee or I pack snacks like raw walnuts, cashews, almonds, and/or macadamia nuts and eat with raw sliced goat or sheep cheese pieces.

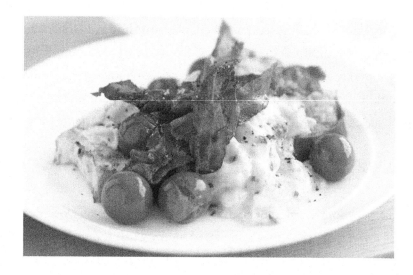

Sample Menus:

Keep in mind to eat when hungry, but not starving. Balance out your macronutrients based on your Metabolic Type test results.

Don't think of your meals as breakfast, lunch, and dinner, rather a meal any time of the day when needed.

You should feel energized about twenty minutes after eating and full for four hours if you ate the right foods for your type.

Sample Menu One

Breakfast:

2-4 scrambled whole eggs topped with sliced avocado, tomatoes, and cooked spinach. Cook eggs with coconut oil at medium heat.

Or

One Shakeology shake mix with water, 1 tablespoon raw nut butter plus add 1 tablespoon MCT and 1-2 tablespoon of raw nuts

Lunch:

4-6 ounces grilled chicken or turkey breast with large leafy spring salad tossed with colorful vegetables, avocado slices topped with 1 teaspoon olive oil and balsamic vinegar

Snack (if hungry):

Vegetable crudités

Measure serving: Raw unsalted almonds, macadamia nuts or cashews with sprinkle of raw unsweetened coconut flakes

Hardboiled egg

Dinner:

4-6 ounces baked salmon or sea bass (wild) cooked with coconut oil or BBQ with lots of vegetables roasted in coconut oil

1 cup plus roasted vegetables cooked with coconut oil topped with 1 tablespoon crushed raw unsalted cashews

Sample Menu Two

Breakfast:

2-3 eggs fried in coconut oil and a slice of protein source (Cook in a pan over medium heat with coconut oil until golden brown on each side) top with fresh pico de gallo and half an avocado

Or

One Shakeology shake with water and ice with MCT oil, spinach, blend in half an avocado.

Lunch:

2-4 ounces Organic chicken sausages or grilled shrimp or scallops (or selects healthy organic grass-fed protein.) Large salad of mixed kale, spinach, and arugula topped with grilled organic vegetables as yellow bell peppers, cucumber, tomatoes, and zucchini slices with a dash of sea salt and pepper, then top with avocado. Lightly sprinkle with raw macadamia nuts and olive oil.

Snack:

2 ½ tablespoons raw unsalted nuts (cashews, walnuts, macadamia, or almonds) with cut-up vegetables such as celery, cucumber, yellow pepper, and/or jicama.

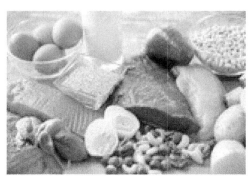

Dinner:

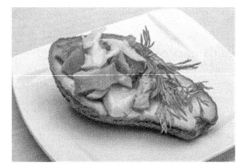

2-6 ounces grilled lean beef or buffalo sirloin (or other lean grass-fed meat) serve with big salad, 2 cups plus of mixed green colorful salad or grilled vegetables. Tossed with lots of shredded organic vegetables such as celery, cucumber, bell peppers, and carrots then toss in one teaspoon olive oil. Or, grill vegetables with coconut oil.

Sample Menu Three

Breakfast:

3 scrambled eggs with 1 cup chopped vegetables and ½ avocado cooked with coconut oil.
Or
One protein shake mixed with a tablespoon of raw almond butter, ice, water and ½ cup coconut milk.

Lunch:

2-4 ounces cod or halibut or other wild fish served over 1-2 cups mixed grilled yellow squash and zucchini slices cooked with coconut oil then topped with one tablespoon raw unsalted cashews or macadamia nuts.

Dinner:

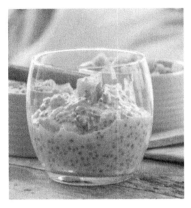

2-4 ounces grilled farm-raised chicken or turkey breast served with 1 cup grilled asparagus topped with one tablespoon crushed raw unsalted walnuts and lemon.

Dessert:

Chia seed pudding mixed with one tablespoon coconut flakes (unsweetened), raw unsalted almond butter and cinnamon. Or one piece of 80% dark chocolate with a teaspoon of raw nut butter.

Sample Menu Four:
Breakfast:
Fat Coffee
Morning Power Smoothie
Chia Seed Pudding
Or
Super Greens Drink: Kale, spinach, celery, cucumber, ginger, and lemon in Omni Blender or Vitamix type of blender.

Lunch:
1-2 sliced hardboiled eggs mixed with roasted spinach and kale topped with sliced avocado, tomatoes, and sprinkled with a few crushed walnuts.

Dinner:
Big, leafy, green salad (kale, spinach, arugula superfoods blend) with clean protein such as grilled shrimp or organic sausages topped with heirloom tomatoes. Mix with olive oil and balsamic vinegar. Sprinkle a little bit of sea salt. Great if eating late.

Some of my favorite Neal meals:

- Bacon served with soft boiled eggs topped with salsa, avocado and full.
- Fat sour cream (if doing dairy).
- Cook blasted Brussels sprouts or broccoli in good source bacon fat (save the fat from your cooking bacon in a side dish) in a big wide wok type of deep saucepan then add bacon pieces and raw walnut pieces.
- Cook zucchini noodles with tomatoes, garlic, yellow peppers, and chicken or protein meat as you prefer.
- Chicken or turkey sausage (Whole Foods) with sauerkraut and stone ground mustard (no sugar added) served with side big green salad greens.
- Super Salad: lots of vegetables including tomatoes, cucumbers, avocado, burrata cheese or goat cheese and butter lettuce topped with olive oil and sea salt plus sprinkle some pumpkin seeds on top.

TIP FOR DINING OUT: ASK FOR WHAT YOU WANT

1. Protein-based: fresh fish (not farm raised) seafood, free-range organic chicken, grass-fed meats

2. Ask for any sauces or dressings on the side. Replace with olive oil and balsamic vinegar

3. Ask for steamed or grilled vegetables instead of bread, rice, pasta, and starchy grains

4. Ask for side of avocado and olive oil when needed

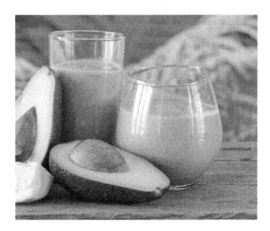

Suggested Snacks:

If you are eating a higher fat food plan, you should be satisfied (full) for 3-4 plus hours. Keep track of emotions, where you are eating, why and level of hunger in your food logs.

1. Green Vegetable Juice: kale, spinach, celery, cucumber, lemon, etc.

2. 2-4 ounces sliced turkey or chicken (grass fed organic) with raw goat or sheep cheese slices

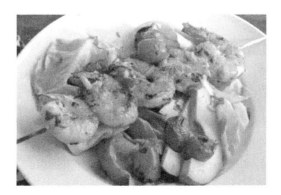

3. ¼ - ½ cup raw nuts (measure serving in baggie) – almonds, cashews, hazelnuts, walnuts, seeds, macadamia nuts
4. Celery sticks with almond butter or try cashew butter
5. Cucumber, celery, red pepper with freshly made guacamole
6. Hardboiled eggs
7. Two ounces grilled chicken breast with four olives
8. Cut up cucumber sticks and cherry tomatoes
9. Shakeology shake with MCT oil or coconut oil with little water (pudding)
10. Grilled or roasted vegetables cooked with coconut oil
11. Mixed salad with tomato, cucumber, spinach, onion, peppers, olive oil and lemon juice
12. Two-four ounces salmon or tuna
13. Chia seed pudding with cocoa nibs or raw nut butter
14. One and a half dark chocolate (80% or greater); Cocoa (non-alkali)
15. One tablespoon almond, cashew, or macadamia butter mixed with one tablespoon coconut oil

Beverages to drink:

- Purified water
- Herbal or Green tea (low caffeine), Jasmine Green tea
- Sparkling or seltzer water with a slice of lemon or lime
- KeVita˙ (Cayenne Lemon is my favorite) less than two grams of sugar

Eliminate for 21-30 days: or consume in moderation:

- ✓ Organic local coffee (1 cup in morning)
- ✓ Alcohol - eliminate for 21-30 days or one drink per week maximum that does not have sugar (i.e., vodka and soda)

Super Power Foods to include in food plan:

1. Coconut oil (organic), MCT oil (see my favorites on website)
2. Vegetables - dark. Green, leafy e. g. chard, kale, spinach; broccoli, Brussels sprouts, cauliflower, tomato, Garlic/onion/ginger, avocado
3. Nuts/nut butter, walnuts, almonds, pecans, peanuts, pumpkin, flax, chia, sesame
4. Cold water fish - salmon (at least once a week)
5. Maca powder

6. Add herbs - cinnamon, pepper (black, cayenne, chili), cinnamon, turmeric
7. Green Tea
8. Dark chocolate (More than 70%)

Green Smoothie Drinks:

Make your own or beware of high sugary drinks, if purchased at the store. Read the ingredients.

- *Clean Green Smoothie*

- *Green Goddess Smoothie*

- *Fight and Repair Smoothie*

The secret to success to transforming the WHOLE you from the inside out is to manage your daily stress or eliminate stressors as eating foods you are sensitive to each day as well as poor digestion.

Remember ...
  ➤ *If STRESS IS ON, then DIGESTION is OFF.*
  ➤ *Every STRESS response is a BLOOD SUGAR response.*
  ➤ *If STRESS is on then the IMMUNE System is depressed.*

Slow down, pause, focus and reset before eating. Deep inhale and a long exhale. Then eat while chewing your food, tasting your food and slowing down the digestion process.

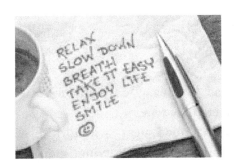

Example of The WHOLESTIC Method Client Plan:

- Focus on low-carb, high fat food plan to heal gut, balance blood sugar and mood
- Meo-energetics Vagal Tone to use pre-meal and pre-bedtime.
- Bed before 9 pm and half hour before sleep time so you can read– get quality sleep by staying off electronics devices pre-bed. Trying reading before and writing gratitude daily journal.
- De-stress by deep breathing with long exhale to "reset" when needed plus gargling, humming and unplugging nature walks will help you slow down, un-wind and reset.

Implement the Leaky Gut Protocol for 30 days:

1. REMOVE foods and factors that damage the gut- sugar, grains, conventional meat, conventional dairy, and GMO foods.
   a. Top toxic exposures to eliminate are tap water, pesticides, NSAIDS and antibiotics.
   b. No commercial dairy
   c. Gluten, grains, wheat
   d. Peanuts
   e. Soy
   f. Sugar

2. REPLACE with healing foods protocol: bone broth, raw cultured dairy, fermented vegetables, coconut products, sprouted seeds, and omega-3 fats.
3. REPAIR with specific supplements
4. REBALANCE with probiotics

https://draxe.com/4-steps-to-heal-leaky-gut-and-autoimmune-disease/
https://draxe.com/7-signs-symptoms-you-have-leaky-gut/

The WHOLESTIC Method:
1. NUTRITION:
   a. Eat real food, low sugar/low carb, moderate protein, and higher healthy fats as per your metabolic type.
   b. Try measuring blood sugar each morning fasted and post meal for 30 days.
   c. Eat when hungry but not starving- should be full 3-4 hours.
   d. Main goal to eat foods that balance blood sugar to reduce insulin surges

e. Try UCAN for longer endurance workouts for slow release carbs/energy
f. Inflammation in body could be related to eating foods you are sensitive to as corn, grains, and sugar.
g. If eating a food that is high carb/sugar, then make sure to balance out blood sugar to avoid insulin surges by eating carbohydrates with fat and protein. HIGH FAT and MODERATE PROTEIN will fill you up for sure!
h. Test microbiome and sensitivities (red/yellow/blue) at www.viome.com and use THEWHOLEATHLETE for your code.

2. EXERCISE:
   a. Strength training 2-3x including mobility drills for hips and spine
   b. Yoga or Pilates Reformer training; for sure use foam roller
   c. Walking outdoor solo time on rest days for ACTIVE Recovery
   d. *Train by heart rate and focus* on building AEROBIC FAT, BURNING ENGINE at MAF heart rate for 80% of your workouts or more.
   e. Add interval (HIIT) strength training 2-3 times per week 20-30 minutes
   f. Tune in the body red flags= alter workouts or take rest day as body tells you!
   g. Set up fitness goals- select event and/or races for extra motivation.

3. STRESS:
   a. Eliminate or reduce coffee/caffeine to less than 2 cups per morning (none after 12 pm)
   b. Deep breathing exercises, walking, meditation, HRV Testing
   c. Reset and recalibrate before eating – deep inhales/longer exhales
   d. Journal- gratitude each night
   e. Measure HEART RATE VARIABILITY daily to track stress, nervous system and over training with Sweetbeat Life app and Bluetooth monitor.

4. SLEEP:
   a. get to bed by 9 pm each night and sleep 7-9 hours per night
   b. Use breathing exercises – counting inhales and longer exhales
   c. Off electronics – iPad, computer, and phones before bed
   d. Be off line two hours before bed or longer: disconnect to connect

5. MOVEMENT: not sitting more than one hour and 10,000 steps per day

6. DIGESTION: leaky gut protocol above and avoiding grains plus sugar (NSNG = no sugar, no grains).

7. HYDRATION: half your body weight in ounces of water per day plus 12-16 oz. for every

8-12 oz. diuretics

8. HAPPINESS: Journal each night before bed – 3 or more things you are grateful for that day.

Download The WHOLESTIC Method daily accountability form available for free on: www.debbiepotts.net.

What is the secret to success on this journey?
- Get your mind right. Be ready to make changes
- Make the commitment to yourself, family, and friends
- Keep the changes simple and stay focused
- One day at a time. Patience is required and trust yourself as this is a new journey and the beginning of a life-long transformation
- N = 1... this will be a self-experiment to discover what works for you as everyone is different not a diet
- We are creating new lifestyle habits
- Positive thinking by eliminating negative self-talk and instead think of your struggles as an area of opportunity

Keep up with your Daily Journal/Accountability Log for at least the 21-Day Challenge or longer. The form can be downloaded for free at www.debbiepotts.net.

Please honestly answer these questions daily.
1. Did you replace a meal a day with our nutritional shake?
    ❑ Yes   ❑ No
2. How was your energy level today?

    _____

    _____

    _____

    _____

    _____

3. How were your cravings for sugar, alcohol, or other vices?

_____

_____

_____

_____

_____

4. Did you eat when you were hungry?
   ❑ Yes   ❑ No

5. How long were you full and satisfied for after you shake or meal?

_____

_____

6. Did you need a snack today because you were hungry?

_____

_____

_____

_____

7. Did you make one green drink per day or buy one without sugar or fruit?
   ❑ Yes   ❑ No

8. Did you sleep seven to nine hours last night?
   ❑ Yes   ❑ No

9. Did you work out today and what did you do?
   ❑ Yes   ❑ No

_____

_____

_____

10. Did you earn over 100 MEPs (MYZONE Effort Points) per workout with your MYZONE belt?

    ❏ Yes   ❏ No

11. Did you drink half your body weight in ounces of water throughout the day? (Remember to drink the Detox drink in the manual: Add a dash of Himalayan salt, apple cider vinegar, plus for added kick add cinnamon or cayenne pepper.)

    ❏ Yes   ❏ No

12. Did you take 10,000 steps today?

    ❏ Yes   ❏ No

13. Did you write in at least three things you are grateful today in your journal this morning or tonight?

    ❏ Yes   ❏ No

14. Send a photo of your meal to our The WHOLESTIC Method Facebook page.

15. Did you achieve your set goals today?

    ❏ Yes   ❏ No

    If not, what are your areas of opportunity? What did you learn about yourself today?

_____

_____

_____

_____

Set goals for tomorrow; because tomorrow is a new day.

STEP #6
PHASE THREE - THE MAINTENANCE PROGRAM

1. Continue eating real food while avoiding gluten/grains, sugar, and bad vegetable oils.
2. Goal: 90/10 rule. Ninety percent (90%) of the time follows the clean eating plan. One cheat card for the twenty-one days, if needed, but I think you can survive twenty-one days with good willpower if you want to change habits and addictive behaviors.
3. Remember this is not a diet, but a new eating lifestyle.

STEP #7
HEALTH QUESTIONNAIRE AND HISTORY

- ➢ New client health history and interview form
- ➢ Nutritional Assessment Questionnaire form and graph
- ➢ Metabolic Typing Form
- ➢ Food Log with symptoms
- ➢ Daily Accountability Report

All forms are available and downloadable at:

www.debbiepotts.net

FOOD CHARTS

Use the following charts for foods to eat, eat in moderation, and those you should avoid altogether.

Healthy Fats – 3-5 servings per day		
Eat Lots	**Eat in Moderation**	**Avoid**
Coconut Oil	Raw Nuts (no peanuts)	Roasted Nuts
Coconut Meat	Raw Seeds	Roasted Seeds
Olive Oil	Almond Butter	Regular Peanut Butter
Macadamia Nut Oil	Palm Oil	Regular Butter
Avocados	Cold Press Flax Oil	Non-Organic Meats
Olives	Bacon	Margarine
Organic Grass-Fed Butter	Mayonnaise	Spreadable Condiments
Organic Yogurt (Full-Fat)	Organic Peanut Butter	Farmed Fish
Ghee	Coconut Ice Cream	Safflower Oil
Free Range Eggs (Yolk)	Dark Chocolate	Sunflower Oil
Grass-fed Beef, Bison,	Pastured bacon fat	Canola Oil
Buffalo, or Lamb	Grain-fed butter	Cottonseed Oil
Sardines, Anchovies, or	Ghee	Commercial Flax Oil
Haddock in Water or Olive	Duck and goose fat	Soy Ice Cream
Oil	Chicken fat	Regular Ice Cream
Wild Salmon, Trout, Tilapia,	Safflower oil	Milk Chocolate
or Flounder	Sunflower oil	Store bought or processed
Triglyceride-Based Fish Oil		salad dressing
Pure Cod Liver Oil		
Grass-fed butter & Ghee		
Pastured egg yolks		
Grass-fed meat fat		
MCT Oil		
Non-GMO soy lecithin		
EVOO		
Chocolate and Cocoa Butter		
Avocado Oil		
Palm Oil		
Vegetables – 3-5 servings per day		
Eat Lots	**Eat in Moderation**	**Avoid**
Sprouts	Sweet Potatoes	Canned Vegetables
Avocados	Yams	Non-organic Vegetables
Olives	Plantains	
Asparagus	Potatoes	Also, avoid if autoimmune
Broccoli	Corn	disease or nightshade
Cauliflower	Peas	sensitivity:

Cabbage	Carrots	
Naturally-Fermented	Celery	Potatoes
Sauerkraut	Cucumber	Tomatoes
Naturally-Fermented Pickles	Squash	Peppers
Bok Choy	Zucchini	Garlic
Collards	Romaine Lettuce	Onions
Swiss Chard	Red Lettuce	Eggplant
Kale	Iceberg Lettuce	
Mustard Greens	Fennel	
Nori (Seaweed)	Radishes	
Organic Greens, powder, or capsules		

Proteins – 2-4 servings per day

Eat	Eat in Moderation	Avoid
Free Range Eggs (with yolk)	Yogurt	Non-Organic Dairy products
Grass-fed Beef, Bison, Buffalo, or Lamb	Cheese	Processed cheese or other pasteurized or cooked dairies (except butter)
Pasture-raised, Organic Pork	Raw cheese from grass-fed cows	
Sardines, Anchovies, or Haddock in water or olive oil	Organic Cottage Cheese	Non-Organic, commercially-produced meat
Wild Salmon, Trout, Tilapia, or Flounder	Naturally preserved or dried meats	Chemically preserved or dried meats
Organic Whey/Casein	Miso, tempeh, tamari, or natty	Protein powders
	Egg protein powder	
	Soaked or sprouted beans/legumes	

Proteins – 2-4 servings per day (continued)		
Eat	**Eat in Moderation**	**Avoid**
Protein Powder Organic Rice/Pea Protein Protein Powder Organic Hemp Protein Powder Organic Yogurt (full-fat)	Raw seeds and nuts Raw nut butter Pastured pork Pastured duck and goose Pastured chicken and turkey Whey protein isolate	Artificial Sweeteners Textured Vegetable Protein Soy Protein Powder Tofu Roasted Seeds and Nuts Roasted Nut Butter Regular or Canned Beans and Legumes High mercury or farmed seafood Factory farmed eggs and meats Wheat protein Beans Cheese and other pasteurized or cooked dairies (except butter)

Non-Vegetable Carbohydrates – one serving per week		
Eat Less	**Eat in Moderation**	**Avoid**
Wild Rice Brown or White Rice Sprouted, Organic Quinoa, Amaranth, or Millet Sprouted Legumes (Beans and Lentils)	Soaked Legumes (Beans and Lentils) Raw Seeds and Nuts Soaked, Organic Quinoa, Amaranth, or Millet Regular Oats Fresh Milled Kamut Wheat Soaked and Sprouted Wheat Products Non-GMO Corn Gluten-free Oats	Canned Legumes Any Regular Wheat Products GMO Corn Roasted Seeds and Nuts Fava Beans Soy Beans Soy Nuts Regular Yogurt Cookies, Biscotti, Scones Crackers Bagels Bread Cereal

Fruit – Limit 1 serving per day or less during Sugar Detox		
Eat with Limits	**Eat in Moderation**	**Avoid**
Apples	Lemons	Canned Fruit
Apricots	Limes	Fruit in Syrup
Bananas	Grapes	Fruit Candy
Berries	Strawberries	Sugar-coated Dried Fruit
Cherries	Dates	Packaged Dried Fruit
Cantaloupe	Figs	
Grapefruit	Natural Dried Fruit	
Kiwi	Fruit Juices	
Mangoes		
Nectarines		
Oranges		
Papayas		
Peaches		
Pears		
Pineapples		
Plum		

Herbs, Spices & Sweeteners – Use when needed		
Add Lots	**Eat in Moderation**	**Avoid**
Cinnamon	Red Pepper	Raw Pollinated Honey
Cloves	Black Pepper	Organic Maple Syrup
All-spice	Fermented Soy Sauce	Natural Fruit Sweeteners
Turmeric	Apple Cider Vinegar	Blackstrap Molasses
Curry	Stevia	Sucanat
Cumin		Truvia
Fennel		Processed Sugar
Star Anise		Candy
Garlic		High-fructose Corn Syrup
Ginger		Regular Honey
		Agave Honey
		Aspartame
		Sucralose
		Acesulfame
		MSG
		Brewer's Yeast
		Xylitol
		Maltitol
		Regular Table Salt

FORMS, CHARTS, LOGS, JOURNALS AND DIARIES

To get any of the forms, charts, logs, journals, and/or diaries listed in this manual and workbook, go to my website and download these forms for free at any time.

www.debbiepotts.net/new-client-forms

These are the forms I will use with you on our The WHOLESTIC Method coaching program:

- Step One: Initial Interview Confidential Client Health Questionnaire
- Step Two: The 3-Day Food Journal
- Step Three: The Nutritional Assessment Questionnaire
- Step Four: Metabolic Type Question
- C.H.E.K. Nutrition in a Nut Shell
- The Eight Forms of Wealth Chart
- The WHOLESTIC Method Daily Accountability Report

ACKNOWLEDGEMENTS

Thank you to those who always inspire me to do more to help inspire millions as well as to those who inspire me to learn more to help be a better coach/trainer/leader.

Of course, I must always acknowledge my amazing, love of my life, best friend, training partner, travel friend and all-in-one husband, Neal Potts, who is always supportive in everything I do.

My coaches, Todd Durkin and Larry Indiviglia.

My Todd Durkin Mastermind Family, for always motivating me to follow my dreams and my BHAG.

My Fitness Forward Studio clients/family, for always keeping me smiling and laughing as well as loving my job. I love the community we have; it's definitely an amazing Fitness Family.

My family for inspiring me to learn more about healthy eating habits for real life.

My mother-in-law, Phyllis Potts, who passed away last year and was the first to introduce me to grain-free cookbooks as well as inspire my awareness of the benefits of coconut oil for memory and diseases, such as Parkinson's, as well as my sister-in-law, Natalie Potts, for all her inspiration on natural healing and nutritional conversations.

And, last, but not least, to all the wonderful guests on my podcast, The WHOLE Athlete, who shared knowledge to help us all become more WHOLESTIC individuals from the inside and out:

Mark Allen

Brock Armstrong

Dr. Josh Axe

Josh Beloff

Angie Check

Paul Chek

Ronda Collier

Todd Durkin

Sally Edwards

Dr. Chad Edwards

Maria Emmerich

Jill Ginsberg

Dina Griffin

Jill Grunewald

MaryLou Harris

Gonzales Helguero

Brad Kearns

Laura Kunces

Geoff Lecovin

Dr. Phil Maffetone

Dr. Amy Meyers

Jimmy Moore

Teri Mosey

Mike Mutzel

Tim Noakes

Nutritional Therapy Association

Jator Pierre

Jonathan Ross

Vinnie Tortorich

Anna Vicino

William Wolcott

ABOUT THE AUTHOR

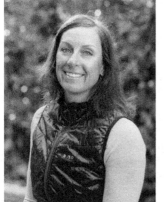

Debbie Potts is the owner, trainer, and coach of a unique personal training and group training boutique private fitness studio in downtown Bellevue, Washington. She has been in the fitness industry for twenty-five years and has continued to learn even more.

Her Fitness Forward Studio offers amazing total body efficient workouts using a variety of tools (or toys.) including free weights, TRX, Rip Trainers, sandbags, kettlebells, medicine balls, slam balls, wall balls and more plus we Pilates mat, yoga, functional strength movements, and sport specific exercises into our workouts.

Debbie's specialties include personal, semi-private and group personal training, mobility training, functional strength training, TRX suspension training, STOTT Pilates, Yoga, Rehab training, Metabolic Testing, C.H.E.K Holistic Lifestyle coaching, and USAT Triathlon coaching. Her next certification is to become a Nutritional Therapy Practitioner. She focuses on coaching clients with The WHOLESTIC Method while training clients on proper form, alignment, and muscle recruitment. Debbie continues to educate her clients the skills how to listen, tune in and focus on their bodies during exercises for the best results -and to avoid injuries. Debbie believes in coaching clients to improve performance for life and sports with her The WHOLESTIC Method. Her coaching programs help clients focus not only on their exercise but also their nutrition, sleep, stress, digestion, hydration, movement, and happiness.

Debbie has been a competitive athlete for most of her life. She has been a top age-group triathlete and runner as well as a fifteen times Ironman finisher, five times Ironman Hawaii World Championship qualifier, and multiple Boston Marathon qualifier. Debbie completed over twenty plus marathons and half marathons. She coaches clients individually on metabolic efficiency, running, trail running, cycling, and triathlon events.

Check out her race results here:

http://www.athlinks.com/athletes/41680626/Profile

Get Connected with Debbie

Text the word 'THEWHOLEATHLETE' to the number 31996 to receive free tips and tricks to transform the WHOLE you from the inside out with The WHOLESTIC Method elements

Find Debbie on Facebook, Instagram, Pinterest, and YouTube for more tips and tricks how to become a WHOLESTIC Athlete by working from the inside out to perform your best in life and sports.

Social Media Connects:
Website: www.debbiepotts.net
Podcast: www.thewholeathletepodcast.com
Facebook: www.facebook.com/fitnessforwardbellevue
Twitter: twitter.com/thewholeathlete
Pinterest: www.pinterest.com/WholesticMethod/
Instagram: www.instagram.com/thewholesticathlete/
YouTube: http://tinyurl.com/DebbieYouTubeList
or https://www.youtube.com/user/FitForwardBellevue

Subscribe to Debbie's podcast, The WHOLE Athlete:
http://tinyurl.com/WholeAthleteiTunes or
http://thewholeathletepodcast.com

Learn more about Debbie's The WHOLESTIC Method coaching:
www.thewholesticmethod.com

Debbie's Practitioners and Peers:
http://kalishwellness.com/
http://www.nourishbalancethrive.com/
http://www.fernlifecenter.com/
http://drgeofflecovin.com/
http://www.chronicconditioncenters.com/exceptional-life-wellness-.html

http://www.sagemed.co/

http://sweetwaterhrv.com/

https://philmaffetone.com/

https://bengreenfieldfitness.com/

http://www.wehlc.com

http://chekinstitute.com/

http://nutritionaltherapy.com/

http://www.markallencoaching.com/

www.skywalkerfitness.ca/

http://bradkearns.com/

DEBBIE POTTS' EDUCATION, TRAINING AND CERTIFICATIONS:

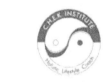

CHEK Holistic Lifestyle Coach

Superhuman Certified Coach

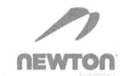

Newton Natural Running Coach

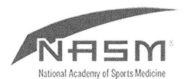

NASM Certified Personal Trainer & CPT Externship Mentor

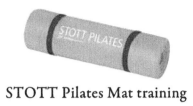

STOTT Pilates Mat training

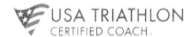

USAT Level One Certified Coach

Yoga Fit and Shakti Yoga training

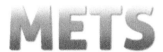

METS: Metabolic Efficiency Training Specialist

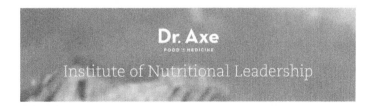

The Institute of Nutritional Leadership with Dr. Josh Axe

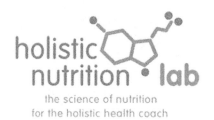

Digestive Intensive

www.holisticnutritionlab.com

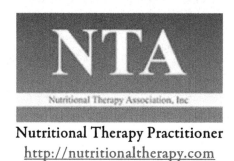

Nutritional Therapy Practitioner

http://nutritionaltherapy.com

Can you help me lose weight?

Debbie also leads a 5-Day Jumpstart Challenge or 21-day Sugar Detox & Reset Challenge for individuals as well as group events and workplaces. Debbie's WHOLESTIC Method coaching style is designed to help clients become healthier versions of them from the inside out to reach peak performance in life and sports.

Debbie coaches clients in person or online, and offers check-in support calls to assist clients in changing eating and lifestyle habits, such as eliminating gluten, commercial dairy, soy, corn, and peanuts (plus limit/cut alcohol and caffeine).

www.thewholesticmethod.com.

What is Debbie's Athletic Background?

Debbie has been a competitive athlete for most of her life. She has been a top age group triathlete and runner, as well as a fifteen-time Ironman finisher, five-time Ironman Hawaii World Championship qualifier, and multiple Boston Marathons qualifiers. She coaches clients individually and online for metabolic efficiency, running, trail running, cycling and triathlon events.

Debbie leads The WHOLESTIC Method programs in person in Bellevue, Washington or online. Start with her Phase One program: The 5-Day Jumpstart Sugar Detox & Reset Challenge then transition into Phase Two: The 21-Day Detox & Reset Challenge. Debbie's goals are to help clients become healthier versions of themselves from the inside out and to become a more efficient fat burning machine.

She offers an online WHOLESTIC Method coaching program starting in 2017 with weekly coaching calls, webinars, and meal ideas as she guides clients through the eight elements to improve health from the inside out. The food plan will include an anti-inflammatory diet for 21 days to eliminate gluten, commercial dairy, soy, corn, and peanuts (plus limit/cut alcohol and caffeine).

Are you ready to push pause and reset your body from the inside out? Transform the WHOLE you with each of The WHOLESTIC Method elements: nutrition, exercise, sleep, stress, movement, digestion/gut health, hydration, and happiness. Discover the new and improved you that is hiding on the inside. You don't know until you find out. Let me know how your journey goes as you choose to take The WHOLESTIC Road. I would love to hear your success stories, wins, ah-has and transformation you have made.

Head to The WHOLESTIC Method Facebook page or send a message on the website www.debbiepotts.net so you can pay-it-forward and inspire others to become the WHOLE Athlete.

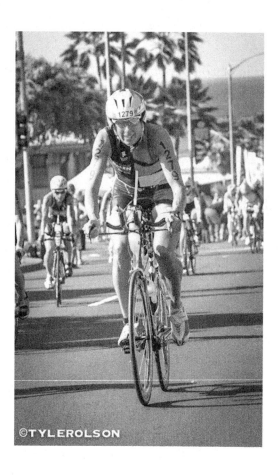

SUGGESTED LINKS AND RESOURCES

- ✓ Lab testing Athlete's Blood testing for detailed lab work (TheWHOLEAthlete for discount code)

- ✓ Microbiome testing by www.Viome.com for gut biome and food allergies (use THEWHOLEATHLETE code)

- ✓ Sweet Beat Life app for heart rate variability and stress monitor

- ✓ Order your MYZONE heart rate monitor and join our community challenges: http://buy.myzone.org/ship/?lang=enUS&voucher=FITFORUS001-3692

- ✓ My favorite Amazon Shopping Page and Biotic Supplements- see links on www.debbiepotts.net

- ✓ Subscribe to my blogs and free books on http://debbiepotts.net

- ✓ Robb Wolf's Paleo Food Matrix - http://www.paleomadeline.com/what-is-paleo/paleo-food-matrix/

- ✓ Sean Croxton's Dark side of Fat Loss link on www.fitnessforwardstudio.com

- ✓ Subscribe to my health and fitness podcast on iTunes or Stitcher Radio to learn more about elements of the WHOLESTIC Method: www.thewholeathletepodcast.com

- ✓ Lots of articles, videos, and blogs on working-in and working-out on http://chekinstitute.com/blog/category/diet/

- ✓ www.nutritionaltherapy.com for articles and updates

- ✓ Ketone Supplement: https://thewholesticmethod.pruvitnow.com

APPENDIX

Here are some notes on MCT Oil from a podcast interview with Brock Armstrong:

- MCT oil benefits include brain health. Feed the brain with ketones which are produced from the MCT oil. The brain will use glucose first then use Ketones if no glucose is available. The brain will use glucose if you have lots of carbohydrates in your diet which change your entire eating strategy to low carb and high fat to avoid damage to your body (eating high fat and high carb = astherocolosis).
- MCT oil are fats found in foods like coconut oil (four types of MCT oil)
- Triglycerides = fat which are needed for transporting
- Increase your healthy fats

Science of Medium-Chain Fatty Acids

MCTS have 6-12 carbon atoms

    (C6, C8, and C10 are also known as Capra Fatty Acids)

1. **C6** = Caproic Acid:
   - Not used as much as unpleasant taste and funny smell
   - Burns the back of the throat and doesn't taste as good
   - May cause disaster pants
2. **C8** = Caprylic Acid:
   - More rapidly absorbed and processed for energy over C12
   - Metabolized quickly - doesn't go through liver to be metabolized
   - Only takes three steps to create ATP (energy for cells) versus sugar that takes 26 steps to create energy
   - Easy way to power the body
   - Takes 18 tablespoons of coconut oil to get = 1 tablespoon of Caprylic acid (direct method)
3. **C10 = Capric Acid**
   - Less rare, 9% of coconut oil made up of Capric acid
   - Longer to break down

- 6 tablespoons of coconut oil to get 1 tablespoon of Capric acid

4. **C12 = Lauric Acid**
   - Biggest part of coconut oil
   - Metabolized by the body almost as long-chain triglycerides
   - Less efficient way to obtain energy than C8 or C10 MCTs
   - Problem is it stops in liver to get broken down for energy so not as quick and direct
   - Unique health benefits: anti-microbial properties. The benefits that may kill off harmful bacteria and viruses
   - C14 and higher are long-chain triglycerides

MCT oil, Coconut Oil, and Ketosis:

1. https://authoritynutrition.com/mct-oil-101/
2. http://draxe.com/caprylic-acid/
3. http://www.coconutketones.com/whatifcure.pdf
4. http://www.coconutketones.com/
5. http://draxe.com/mct-oil/

Contact Debbie Potts for more information via www.debbiepotts.net, and follow on social media.

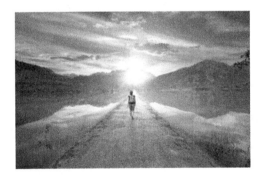